King Of

CW01498928

Tom Gray

chipmunkapublishing
the mental health publisher

Tom Gray

All rights reserved, no part of this publication may be reproduced by any means, electronic, mechanical photocopying, documentary, film or in any other format without prior written permission of the publisher.

Published by
Chipmunkapublishing
United Kingdom

http://www.chipmunkapublishing.com

Copyright © 2014 Thomas A. Gray

ISBN   978-1-78382-093-1

Front cover photograph: Trafford Photography
Back cover photograph: Thomas J Simons Photographic Plc
Back cover photo edit: Fraser Blakemore Design Co

Chipmunkapublishing gratefully acknowledge the support of Arts Council England.

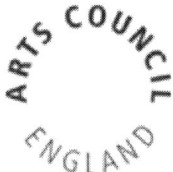

IN THIS WORLD THERE IS NO BLACK OR WHITE

JUST A GRAY AREA

Tom Gray

KING OF THE WORLD

It's hard to put into words the unimaginable darkness that can descend upon your life in such as short amount of time. It feels like the lights have been switched off in your world and the sun has set for the very last time. This decent into oblivion is beyond description, the fear that runs through your core is like something you have never felt before. You try to fight against this black hole that you are being dragged into but you cannot. You are buried deep in the void, a perpetual abyss far beyond human imagination. They say pain doesn't last forever but here it does. You know there is no way of being set free, the feeling of despair, loneliness and dread consumes every fibre of your being and distinguishes any fraction of hope left within you. Life becomes a waiting game, you know your purpose on this earth is no more and you are now an unwanted item that is waiting to be disposed of. Although you know the end is approaching you cannot find peace within yourself, your time on this world may be over but your fears of your next destination are so powerful that you cling on to this life with all you have. There is nothing left inside you except survival but you know you cannot survive forever and soon the day will come when you depart this life and move onto the next.

This isn't just a bad day and despite popular belief you can't pull yourself together and simply snap out of it. Sometimes behind the biggest of smiles hides the deepest of sadness. Inside you are slowing dying and you simply feel like no one will ever understand or make things better.

Contrary the feeling of immense power that consumes your body and mind is impossible to quantify. Everything that you ever dreamed of is now becoming a reality. You have no fear of anybody or anything, your time has come to change the world for the better.

Welcome to the world of Bi-Polar. There is no choice with this illness or any other mental illness, you cannot opt out. Unfortunately you've been handed a life sentence with no chance of payroll.

I. 50 PENCE

I'm sat writing this after spending nearly 3 months inside a psychiatric hospital; how can an average lad from Sheffield go from living a normal life to 2 suicide attempts and 3 hospital admissions? We may never know why this illness came to nearly ending my life but it will be interesting to know whether or not any of the choices I made or the way I conducted myself had any impact on my life.

People ask me will this book help them understand why I became unwell, if I'm being honest I don't think it will. This is because I feel there isn't reason. Well not one I can come up with at this moment in time. I guess it's just like a physical illness, they just occur and get treated accordingly. Just like cancer does not target a specific person neither does mental illness. What I can tell you is there are ways in which you can conduct your life which can reduce the chances of any future occurrences. Much research has been done relating to the chemicals in your brain, when these become unbalanced it causes changes in how your mind works. Certain drugs are designed to alter the chemicals in your brain such as Dopamine and Serotonin, when there are deficiencies or abundances then that's where the problems can occur. Luckily for me by adding chemicals into my brain, the imbalances become more stable and 'normal' life can resume. As for why they became imbalanced in the first place I don't know. Why didn't one of my other friends become unbalanced or my brother? I don't know that either. Maybe one day we will find out but for now we will just keep learning.

I grew up in a small village called Aston which is located on the border between Sheffield and Rotherham. If people ask where I'm from I always say Sheffield. My Dad Mark is Rotherham through and through compared with my Mum Tracie who was brought up in the posh side of Sheffield, Dore.

Both my Grandad's were butchers, as well as numerous past generations who were all butchers. My maternal Great Grandfather was a fishmonger and he and other relations all worked at some point in Castle Market together. Grandad Don had butchers shops in Rotherham town centre and others on the outskirts. He had great success in his early days and became very established, he and my Nannan Jean had 5 children. Don used to have a passion for nice cars and even used to be a racing driver at one time, his brother used to be a gangster in Rotherham in the Moony Gang and I'm told he used to drive a Rolls Royce. My Grandad was a quiet man but he used to take me to play snooker and I always enjoyed that. Unfortunately my Grandad died of a stroke a number of years ago and his last years were not as fulfilling as his earlier years. Just before I was born my Dad and my Grandad Malcolm had bought a shop in Thurcroft, Rotherham and my Dad is Managing Director of the shop to this day and it is now in its 27th year which is an achievement in itself given certain external factors, it is a success that he doesn't give himself enough credit for. Most other butchers would not have made it through. Malcolm semi-retired and co-owned a caravan site in Runswick Bay near Whitby which he has since sold and now enjoys retirement in a small village just outside Whitby with his partner Margaret who has been a fantastic support especially in recent years. Grandad Malcolm is a fantastic man and I really enjoy going to see him in Whitby, he has a very good sense of humour. Although I don't see him a great deal, it's about quality time not quantity of time and for that I am very lucky. He too loves his motor cars and is well known for his frequent change of vehicle, my Grandmama would often tell me how he would change cars more than his underpants. He and my Grandmama Sue are divorced but had fantastic success in their early days, his business flourished and did really well and they had 2 amazing children, one of course is my mother and the other is my uncle and close friend Mark. While were on the subject my Grandmama decided before my birth that she would not be called 'Grandma' but instead 'Grandmama'. This was because it sounded better and less common, nobody at thought it would work but all 4 of her Grandchildren obeyed this command. I will however refer to her from this point as Grandma. My uncle is alternative to say the least, I mean that in the greatest of ways. He has a fantastic outlook on life and I too have tried to extract some of his concepts and merge them into my own ideals. He has a daughter, Nuala who is half Danish and half English and is a credit to him.

I am the oldest child of three, with a younger brother called Alex who is 4 years younger than me and a sister, Christie who is 6 years younger than me. My brother is totally opposite to me, he does what he wants and doesn't worry too much about what people think. That may sound harsh but it's not a criticism as he does it in a nice way. I on the other hand worry too much about what people think and try to please everyone before myself. Now I'm not saying I'm a saint and he isn't but what I'm trying to say is we have two different approaches on life. Now he hasn't been sectioned or lost his marbles and has a great job and his own little family, so I guess the proofs in the pudding. However what suits one doesn't necessary suit another. He is a fantastic person and has a heart of gold, extremely intelligent and in his day very good with the ladies. I have a heart of gold but not the last two so I don't feel the attributes were distributed evenly upon our creations. I remember one time going to the dentist in Kimberworth Park, I was probably about 11. The dentist looked in my mouth and said I that I need a brace and 4 teeth removing due to over crowding. Of course I was gutted, and then it was Alex's turn. He was in the chair about 20 seconds 'lovely looking teeth Alex no work is required here'. That kind of sums it up. Alex is now very settled with his girlfriend Nicole, they have been going out for around 4 years and have a house together in nearby Handsworth. Nicole is fantastic and the two of them are really well suited. She keeps him in check and that is good for him.

Then there's my sister Christie. Just like her mother and grandmother, very strong and wise. She's kind of got the mix right between me and Alex. She does what she wants but in a better way that doesn't rub people up the wrong way. Christie is very driven and I feel she will do very well in what she does in the coming years. Not really a bad word to say, but like most women, moody. But the best ones are I guess. Me and my Mum often joke that she has Bi-Polar and not me. Christie and her partner James are very settled and he fits very well into our family and from the outside looking in makes her very happy which is all I wish for really.

As a child I always felt out of place somehow, most of my parent's friend's children were younger and I used to find it difficult to mix in with them. I would often find myself either on my own or with my parents and their friends. I didn't belong with either group and would often feel very outcast. That feeling of never fitting in kind of followed me throughout my life and still does even to this day but nowhere near as much as it did, however I have learned good coping strategies which help a lot. Family life was very normal really, of course I fell out with my parents over the years but nothing that I would deem as being abnormal. I have a very close relationship with my Grandma who has been a great support especially in tough times not only for me but also my family. She's also been there for the good times too. She would always take us out for tea when we were young and wouldn't let us wear jeans to go out and we had to wear 'proper' trousers. I didn't like that but of course I enjoyed going out with her so made a compromise. My Grandma told me that when Alex was born she had asked me when it would be a good idea for us to bring him out with us for tea and I apparently replied with "ok but when he's nine"! I was very fortunate to have a Great Gran and she was certainly Great. She used to come on two buses from Totley over to Aston to see us every week. She would bring with her loads of goodies which I had requested, namely vanilla slices, Eccles cakes and lots of chocolate, Lindt to be precise. I was very close to my Gran and I used to talk to her a lot, she was like a best friend more than anything. She used to play games such as patience and pairs with me and I always used to look forward to Mondays and Tuesdays. She would sleep in my room on a settee bed and I would spend ages making it all comfy for her with loads of cushions and even a little light. She loved snooker and more importantly loved Jimmy White, it would have been great for her to meet him. I decided to buy us some tickets and I took her to The Crucible Theatre to watch the World Championship Snooker and she loved it. I cherished every moment I spent with her as I knew she would not be around forever and once I got my scooter I used to go over frequently to give something back for all the things she had done for me as by that time she wasn't able to come and see us. Ever since I was a young teenager all I wanted to do was get a car and take my Gran home in it, and my wish came true. I used to take her home on Tuesdays after passing my test. My Gran reminded me of the Queen Mother and she loved the royals, we would watch the Queens speech every Christmas Day. She moved over to Aughton, which is next to Aston eventually and we all helped her move, I did loads of work in the garden as I wanted it to be as nice as possible for her. After everything she had given me over the years it was the least I could do. She didn't stay very long in her bungalow and her health deteriorated rather quickly.

My Gran is now 94 years old but unfortunately has Dementia. She is in a nursing home in Rotherham where she receives great care, the whole issue brings great sadness to my Grandma (her daughter) as we all know she would just love to 'float away' (her words) but that unfortunately has not happened. I have fond memories of my Great Gran and often float of into my own world thinking of them and I also blame her for my ridiculously sweet tooth!

I went to Aughton Nursery and then onto school at Aston Hall Junior and Infant, which was conveniently located on my estate and was in walking distance, it was known as the 50p School as it was shaped like a 50p piece. I had a good set of friends but felt very unsure of myself. I thought that no one wanted to be my friend and again lacked in self-confidence. I guess from the outside looking in people would see a totally different picture but for me I had a different truth, a truth much darker than reality. It's hard to describe how I felt in those days, I think I just wasn't happy. This of course isn't a blanket emotion. I just wanted to be more popular or just to feel nicer inside. I remember not been able to sleep at school and one of my best friends at the time, James (Jnr school James), also didn't. He had spoken to his Dad about this and he said "well if you can't sleep tonight, don't worry as you'll sleep tomorrow night". It helped a lot as once you take the worry out of not sleeping you more often than not do fall asleep. Me and James had some fantastic times, he had a go kart and we used to ride down his road. We did this for years and never got bored. My friendship with James drifted as we came to the end of junior school.

There were other happier times at junior school, for instance my good friend Tom and I had our very own 'two table' in Year 4 which was Mr Rodison's class. Rodison was a fantastic pianist and used to play all the music for us to sing along too. When he got angry he used to slam a book so hard on the table all the birds in the playground would fly away.

Me and Tom used to basically piss about all the time, laughing and joking all day or until the teacher told us to stop but my laughing was so uncontrollable that I couldn't stop which would get me into trouble, Tom's a funny kid and his antics would get me into more trouble further down the line. There were other good times at junior school but my overriding memory was not feeling good enough and that something was amiss.

On this one occasion it was Richard's birthday another good friend of mine from junior school, as kids the parties usually consisted of hiring out a parish hall and eating sandwiches and space raiders or if we were lucky bowling. But no not Richard, he rented out a massive inflatable laser quest for us all to play in. It was huge and it spread over one entire lawn. Us lot often went up to Richard's to play on his quad bike or run around the barn jumping on bales of hey. There was always something exciting going on up there and it just kinds of summarises how us kids in Aston roll. Aston is no Essex admittedly but its got something about it that no other place has, I'm not sure if it's the high diversity of people or it's just because its home. I know one thing for sure though us lot have more fun than those wannabes down South. Plus we'd probably win if we had a fight. The Only Way is Aston would be a hit, starring yours truly of course.

On a separate time at Richard's some of his Mum's friends were round who were police officers. It was decided, for some unbeknown reason, to ask the police officers if they would pretend to arrest me. Now I don't think there was any malice intended but for the life of me I still cannot understand why they did this. The end result was I burst into tears and was totally petrified. I was only 10 or so. Richard still finds it amusing and doesn't seem to quite fathom why I was so frightened. Ever since then I have always had a feeling in the back of my mind that somebody would take me away.

My Year 6 teacher Mr Rowan told me I had a good sense of humour but didn't know when to stop, looking back I can totally agree with him. There was on this one occasion the 'berry incident' this basically involved our little gang chucking berries at this poor lad's house. There were about five of us there, the end result was this lad's parents came round to my mates house to basically tell us off. Well silence fell as we were getting a good telling off but I started giggling so much so that Kevin, Tom's Dad, had to intervene but unfortunately this meant that I laughed even more to the point of Kevin getting increasingly cross with me. My problem of laughing at inconvenient times still sticks with me today although much less frequent than it used to be.

When I look back on my life I feel very blessed with the childhood I had. Most of the problems were created within me, some kids have an awful childhood whether it be bullying, abuse or bad parenting, I had none of that. My Mum worked as a secretary but from home, this meant we benefitted from having a parent there for us full time. My Mum would work whilst we were at school and she would more often than not work until the early hours of the morning. My Mum has never really been career minded but if she was she would more than likely be running the NHS by now.

My Dads over riding advice to me as a child was "don't become a butcher". This was mainly due to the hard times he has had since taking the shop. There was BSE, foot and mouth plus the mass takeover from supermarkets. In addition to this the pit closed in Thurcroft as well as other local services like the bank and the fruit and veg shop which all led to a major downturn in the local economy. To top it off the council embarked on the most ridiculous parking scheme on the shop fronts which means no bugger can get parked even if they wanted to visit the shop. He has done an amazing job in supporting his family given the situation he's in, we live in a lovely house and go on great holidays but it's not been easy and certainly isn't getting any easier. I think his business struggles over the years have had a negative impact upon his life. I'm not totally sure as it's not something that is spoken about. He has recently started a new venture doing home deliveries and advertises via text and Facebook and is having reasonable success with this.

I used to help in the shop at Christmas sometimes with my Grandad, Don. I once remember been in the shop and my granddad was gutting a Turkey. This bloke came in and was telling my Dad all about his new car, blabbering on for ages. My granddad just lifted his head up and said "I don't know what all the fuss is about it's only a Toyota" then put his head back down and carried on.

As I'm writing this there is the horsemeat scandal, which you would think would encourage punters into the shop however they cannot get parked!! There hasn't really been an increase in trade probably due to the fact no one can really afford an alternative to the cheap meat products they were originally buying plus people are uneducated and don't know what good food is.

A couple of years ago I did arrange a mass leaflet campaign as I had watched the television programme The Apprentice twice and thought I could turn my Dad's shop into some kind of gold mine. We delivered 5000 leaflets in the local area but unfortunately we only yielded a few extra customers but it was worth a try.

From the age of 14 I started gardening for a select number of clients in the Aston and Swallownest area. I used to charge £5 per hour and I probably had 4 clients, so probably netted £20 on a good week (weather depending of course). I used to love it and built up quite a good relationship with all my clients and from that age I knew I could build bonds with people. My favourite client was a lady called Lilian and we still keep in touch now nearly 15 years down the line, I don't see her as much as I used to but still call in now and then and up until recently washed her car. I learned a lot about life from her and she is a true gem. I once even rode around the estate on her mobility scooter which was a laugh. The gardening continued and in fairness never really went away I still get the odd call and sometimes put in a special appearance. In addition to the relatively good financial rewards I used to receive I also got the odd Date and Walnut cake which used to go down a treat. That's the only date I was ever close to getting. In addition to my Gardening I used to wash my Dads 3 series BMW Coupe religiously every Saturday, I used to clean it inside and out and polished it. I hoped that by washing the car every week my Dad would give it to me when I passed my test. The truth is my Dad would have done if he could have afforded to replace it but anyway my parents always went around in a nice shining car.

So from an early age I always used to keep busy and wanted to be out and about, as I said earlier I was fairly confident selling my services to the elderly however once an old man chased me down his driveway for offering my gardening services (I tried a door to door campaign) and he came close to whacking me with his stick! He was offended that I suggested his garden needed improving which was a fair comment in hindsight.

However, when it came to mixing with my peers I was always less confident. I would often think I was the least respected or liked in a group. This didn't create too much bother for me, I used to wish I was more liked for sure but there were no major signs of any problems. These feelings of not being popular continued throughout my school life. I was very happy at secondary school and had a fantastic network of friends, I would say I took a back seat at school and didn't try to be anyone I wasn't. I just accepted that I wasn't an alpha male and just got on with life, this positive 'laissez a faire' attitude however unfortunately didn't last forever. I made a new friend in secondary school and that was Sam, he became one of my best mates and still remains so today. Sam's unique and doesn't have much fear. He's a good lad to have on your side, he provided me endless entertainment and he was in a lot of my classes, he used to wind the teachers up something chronic. We used to see a lot of each other outside of school and I would more often than not be around at his house or in his shed whilst he was mending his BMX. Sam was an exceptional athlete and competed for the English schools championship throwing Javelin's. He could throw things for miles, never underestimate Sam's throwing capacity and he is so strong, he once lifted a massive granite work top unaided from his van to somebody's house. He was a fantastic mate growing up and only added to my childhood. Sam's journey hasn't been easy over the years for one reason or another but he's overcome more obstacles than most to get to where he is today. He is an invaluable member of the gang and ranks very highly.

I had a very happy childhood, I worked hard both in and out of school but I was always the quiet one in a group and to be fair I still am fairly reserved now.

2. WINDMILL MAN

My pals and I created a gang, we were the OTWC which stands for On Two Wheels Crew. We all were into our push bikes, my Mum and Dad bought me a Giant Boulder Shock for Christmas and I had this bike until I went to University. Whilst I was at Uni I forgot to chain the bike up, well I did chain it up but I failed to incorporate the bike in the fastening which basically meant my bike was not chained up which resulted in the theft of my beloved Giant. I had upgraded every single part of the bike and it stood me at a lot of money. This paved the way for my Specialised P3 which was a good bike for jumping, but I couldn't jump so it was pointless me having such a bike. I gave this bike to my brother and he was chuffed to bits with it however I needed some cash and sold it to some marine of eBay. He still gets upset about that now and one day I'll buy him a bike. I have recently bought a Giant Trance which is an enduro bike but I also can't ride enduro so again this was another one of my pointless purchases. My mate Richard always laughs at me because I told him it was an investment, I thought I would save money going to the gym however I never ride the bike so I'm well over a grand worse off plus I joined the gym anyway. I'm just getting back into it now and my fitness levels are increasing. We try to head off into the peaks and go on some good descents plus me and Tom had the most amazing day at Whinlatter in the Lakes. The natural highs are the greatest these days.

There was about 12 of us in the OTWC all roaming the streets, we never really got into too much bother, well I didn't. We had the odd chase and had a few meetings with the local police establishment but nothing to write home about. We had a lot of fun in what then was a building site called Aston Manor, one day Sam decided to take a dumper truck for a ride as we had a magic key for it. He got into a bit of bother for that, Sam was the one who had the balls in the group. We were good kids just enjoying life at the time. As I look back we had no worries, we all had each other, our bikes and our dreams nothing we thought could ever get in the way. Me and Tom set up another organisation, this was known as the BIA which stands for Brother is Arms after the fantastic song by Dire Straights that Tom's Dad Kevin used to listen too. You will be pleased to know that this organisation still operates to this day however only on light duties.

I did have one bit of bother at school and I suppose looking back at it was bullying. It was a kid called Woody, he was the year below me and was smaller than me but he scared the crap out of me. He used to wait for me on the bus, a bus which went nowhere near his house. He used to make gestures with his fists and he used to watch where I went for dinner. He wanted to fight me but I didn't want to fight him. He just had so much confidence, one time he started on me in the English block at school and my school friend Lee jumped in and saved me. A week or so passed and Richard told my Mum and Dad about the difficulties I was having and they informed the teachers. He tried again to have a fight with me - I was walking back from break along the South corridor but this time I was ready for him and this time I fought back. I had a rucksack on my shoulders and I just went at him like a man possessed chucking my arms all over the place, I gave him a good hiding that day and everyone was cheering because they all knew how he was making my life hell. I didn't have any more problems from him after that day and was known as the windmill man due to my punching technique.

At the age of 16 my Dad bought me my first scooter, an Italjet Formula 50. He thought it would be great for me to get to and from jobs and to help me earn a few extra quid. I was the first one to get a scooter and before I knew it there were about 15 of us all buzzing about like a swarm of bees. We used to go everywhere in them from freezing our knackers off in winter to riding in just shorts on a nice sunny summers day. Again we all had no worries, they only worry we had was getting girlfriends! I speak for myself but I can also include a few of my close friends in this, we were all hopeless. I was the worst, I just seemed to frighten them all away. I was like the leading actor in the InBetweeners TV show. I don't know how I managed to repel women, I tried different haircuts, after shaves and tactics but nothing seemed to work. In the end I took the view that I would never get a girlfriend.

In addition to my part time gardening I managed to get a part time job working in a Petrol Station in a nearby village called Whiston, I went there for a 3 week work experience placement in Year 9 and they kept me on. The owner of the shop, Peter, was an old friend of my Dads. I had a fantastic five years employment there and learned many lessons in life. I also was lucky enough to work with Christine and Diane. Christine was a lovely women and I built up a very good relationship up with her, she would open and close the shop up 7 days a week in addition to working part time at John Lewis, she was an absolute trooper. Peter was a good bloke deep down and I have a lot of respect for him, he taught me some good things about business and life I suppose. He did however have a short temper and if I wasn't doing my job right he'd let me know.

Every Saturday he would bring me a massive bacon sandwich he had made, and I mean it was massive. Other times he would bring me my favourite pizza which was Tropicana from his favourite pizza place but he always made them add loads of hot chillis. They really looked after me, it was a family business and they made me feel like part of the family. I had a lot of fun with Peter on those Saturdays. I also used to valet his car every week. Unfortunately Peter and I fell out after I got back from travelling due to an arrangement we had, I guess it was a miss communication. I believed that he said I could use his garage for free (of course I was going to compensate him in some way) however upon my return he told me via text that I owed him £1.50 per day. This over a year is a considerable amount of money to find. My Mum wrote him a cheque but he never cashed it. Time however is a good healer and we speak again now if only to say hello.

While I was at junior school we had a new person join the school called Ben and he played ice hockey. He was allowed to finish early one day a week to go and play, so after a few months of Ben leaving early I decided I wanted to finish early from school so started to play ice hockey. This however did not accomplish the goal of finishing early as I wasn't allowed too. I did however play ice hockey for a number of years at Kingston upon Hull, for the River Rats and I used to train 3 times a week up in Hull with matches on a Sunday. My Mum and Dad shared the driving from Hull which must have been very onerous and costly. Even when I was playing Ice hockey I felt as if I wasn't good enough and lacked that self-confidence. It's hard to give an explanation as to why I had low self-esteem but it had significant roles in my life in certain situations. My lack of self-confidence was at its greatest in group situations.

Shortly after Ben joined our school he kindly informed me that I was the funniest person he'd ever met. This was a very nice thing to say, it later turned that he had never actually met anybody else before. Ben and I spent a lot of time of the road playing as he too lived on Woodpecker. We have a grass banking at the bottom of our street and we thought it would be a good idea to do grass sledging one day in summer. Well it doesn't work so don't bother trying it. Some days we would throw water bombs at cars from the top of the banking and hide behind the Green electric box. Often cars would stop and we would have to make a swift exit.

I played many sports before and after ice hockey and all finished the same way - by me quitting. I never felt as though I was good enough mainly because I wanted to be the best and if I couldn't be the best then nothing else was good enough. I missed out because being part of a time and feeling needed must add a lot to a child's life growing up.

On reflection, we boys did have a fantastic life; my insecurities disappeared for the most of my time at Aston Comprehensive however they did seem to return in sixth form but I will get onto that later. So the OTWC was in full operation and we used to get up to all sorts, we used to ride everywhere. We were all fortunate as none of us seemed to get much homework, so with all that riding we were all fit as fleas. Towards the end of my secondary education everyone else at school seemed to be out drinking and smoking, we however were just riding about tormenting people on the park. I remember one occasion when one of our group (who will remain unnamed) pinched a massive rocket from the local Cricket Club. We were all running and one of our lot managed to get a piece of drain pipe, so we waited a few hours then as the bonfire night celebrations were coming to an end we set our massive rocket back to the Cricket Club. It looked like something from a war documentary, this rocket set off very low and it dipped then exploded right across them. It was perfect.

Events like this were common place throughout the time period at Aston Comprehensive. I was, I'd say, a popular lad and had many friends. I was separated from Tom when we went to Comp probably due to my poor behaviour with him throughout primary school. It was probably a good thing really in hindsight and I went up to Comp with Ben and another lad. My self-esteem, as I remember, wasn't as low as it had been while at primary school or in fact during my time in sixth form. Been separated from Tom was good in a way as it allowed me to establish myself and create new friendships which I probably wouldn't have done otherwise.

I had an ambition to become a fighter pilot in about year 9 so I joined the Mosborough 860 Air Cadet Squadron, I probably attended the air cadets for about 2 years or so, I even stopped getting hay fever tablets from the doctors as I knew you couldn't become a pilot if you had hay fever. I went along to the air cadets every Tuesday and Thursday with Aidan, Ben and Joe, overall it was very good, I went to a remembrance Sunday parade which was very fulfilling and moving and also did some bag packing at Sainsburys! We used to do shooting and there were camps in the summer but I never had the bottle to attend. I was lucky enough to go flying and I had such an amazing experience, I did all the acrobats and the pilot even let me do a loop the loop. We even flew upside down over York Minster. I have been very lucky along the way with the things I have seen and done. I left the Air Cadets as I was more interested in piloting my pushbike along the streets of Aston and the surrounding suburbs plus Tom called it Air Fagots which he still finds amusing today.

I grew up with a good friend called Aidan who was one of my best friends when I was young. Basically my Mum and Aidan's Mum met whilst they were in hospital giving birth (not actually at the birth but in the hospital). We had a great friendship and we went on a few holidays most of which I was too young to remember. We had some great times together and used to get up to a few little tricks. We used to pretend we were on Men Behaving Badly and we used to drink our cans of shandy bass then throw them behind us like they did on the show. He also had a quad bike and we used to go on missions and I used to be the co-driver on the back! We had some great times, he's a great kid but we grew apart and he went off in a different direction after school. I had and still have a lot of respect for Aidan. He's got himself a nice girlfriend and a house and I have nothing but good wishes for them.

Aston Comprehensive school was very fulfilling I remember taking a back seat and never wanted to be the centre of attention, this however changed later on. Our class 7H had some very interesting characters in it and I had no chance entertaining the class when there were such personalities. I think our class was one of the naughtiest classes with the likes of Tom (7H Tom), Shaun, Carl, James, Fraser and Lee. They used to provide some quality entertainment but we must have been a nightmare for the teachers. Our form teacher left and she was replaced with another who unfortunately couldn't control us and he also left our class to somebody else.

I met a good friend at comp called John, John originally was a member of the infamous Beighton Massive who members of the OTWC have had dealings with over the years. It was funny how we met. Our class was queuing up for double Geography and I saw John who I didn't really know and he was eating a pack of chocolate digestives. Anyway for some strange reason I walked up to him and asked him for one. Well John went crazy at me and was shouting and I think he even kicked me. I couldn't believe it. Anyway it calmed down and later I went up to John for a chat as I felt really guilty. John had had some really bad news and I at the time didn't know this. So I felt rotten about the whole situation. So I tried chatting with him to resolve the bad tension. Over the next few weeks I became fantastic friends with John and since the digestive incident he became one of my closet friend in the early years at Aston Comprehensive. So if you've got no friends and you see someone eating a pack of biscuits, simply just ask for one.

I used to take part in a variety of sports for example cricket, football and rugby and I was hopeless at all of them. I didn't used to dare tackle anybody at rugby in case I got hurt, I was a real sissy. But I always turned up and gave it a go, but once however I realised I wasn't any good or that I wasn't ever going to be the best then I'd pack it in. Cricket was great and I think I enjoyed it the most, mainly because you just stand there or smash a ball as hard as you can but seriously it's a great sport. Aston Cricket Club was lovely and in a nice setting which helped. I once got 3 wickets in a game which was good, my Great Grandad did this and got a medal, I thought I would but later found out you have to get the wickets in a row. I think if I had a son I'd guide him in the direction of cricket because you're with all your mates and they have afternoon tea. Plus there were some top quality lads who played.

That pattern of behaviour i.e. quitting has been with me throughout my life. In terms of grades I did pretty well in my exams, I got 5 C's, 3 B's and 3 A's. I was chuffed with my grades and I still to this day can't believe how I got a C in French, my French teachers used to laugh when I spoke in my lousy French accent. I missed my old junior school mates who were in a separate part of the year to me but it allowed me to make new friends and flourish. One friend who I made in year 10 was called Leila, she was a lovely girl and still is although I don't have a great deal of contact with her but that's my fault I guess. She would often get me into trouble for talking or not paying attention. She was a cracking lass and we had a lot of fun in those Science classes and we built up a very good relationship and people would often think we were together. I was told if I didn't spend as much time talking to Leila then I would have the ability to do well, but when your 15/16 you're more interested in talking to girls. I didn't speak to that many girls, I was and still am very shy when it comes to the opposite sex and I'm even worse if I fancy them a bit! So I had a great relationship with Leila and also made some other great friends. I was very lucky in many ways with school, I had bad times, a few people used to call me gay and tease me a bit, at one point I thought I must be gay because these people are saying it all the time. But that didn't last very long in all fairness and it didn't bother me too much. Some people have it really tough in school and life isn't much fun but I wasn't one of them.

During the early days in comprehensive I made good friends with a lad called Fraser who lived at the top of my estate. I had some fantastic times with Fraser and by spending time with him it opened up my horizons and made me look at life from a different perspective, he's a few years older than me so knew a lot more about life that I therefore he could pass on some of his wisdom to me. He was well into his computer and knew a lot about the world of technology. Around this time we met a load of girls from Kiveton and we would always go and see them together.

In year 10 me and Tom were in the same business studies class and we carried on from where we left off back on the two table in year 4. There are some people in life who you just have fun with no matter where you are or what you're doing and Tom is one of those people. Once again I was getting in trouble and we of course had to be split up. We were becoming more mates again after 3 or 4 years of being apart and we spent an increasing amount of time together outside of school. He was in my Maths class which he still finds strange given his capacity for Maths or Math as he calls it. You know your cleaver when you call it Math. I was very pleased when Tom invited me to go with him and his parents to Alcudia in Majorca. We had an absolute ball over there and got up to some right mischief. We fell in love with these two girls, one was from Cumbria and we called her twinny pink (pink bikini) and the other was from Cardiff and we called her twinny Wales. I don't think they had the same feelings for us and to this day that is still one of my most enjoyable holidays. We did all sorts, we climbed a mountain next to the resort which was very high and we even stole a bicycle buggy, you know the ones the chuckle brothers used to have. We went all over the place and used to offer lifts out to attractive females.

3. THE GT

I completed my full time education in the summer of 2003, on results day Tom, my other friend Chad and I all went into Derbyshire on our scooters. I was buzzing that day, the sun was shining, I was out with my mates and I had just got some fantastic grades. The whole world was at my finger tips and I could achieve whatever I wanted. I had no worries what so ever and everything was just perfect. At the time you don't appreciate enough how good things were, it's only when you look back that you totally appreciate how fantastic life was. At this point in my life I still wasn't drinking and maybe that had a significant impact on how I felt at the time.

My first car was a White 1991 VW Polo 1.0 Mk3, it only had 4 gears but it looked the part and only cost £500. It was a pimp mobile, you know the ones, blacked out windows, big exhaust and when I'd finished with it a big sound system. My uncle Mark once took some students mountaineering from my school and he asked if they knew me to which they responded "yeah he's a rude boy". – I guess I was. I got my car before my driving licence, which meant I could go out with my parents before I obtained my licence. I remember going out with my Mum one time and after about a mile she made me stop the car so I could wind my seat back up to a more acceptable level, wind my window up so I couldn't have my arm out and finally turn down the music. It was the ultimate piece of kit but I would have to wait until I passed my driving test before I could go cruising.

I passed my test in August 2004 and we went on a road trip to Skegness that night which was one of our favourite places to go at the time. It was like a mini adventure, the roads were fantastic but it was a killer setting off for home at 2am, plenty of Red Bull was required. I had wanted to drive so badly for such a long time that to finally be driving was like all my dreams had come true. I even purchased a private number plate which was G2AY T, everyone said it looked like GAY T so I never transferred it onto my new car. This again is another example of how one of my good ideas turns around and bites me on the backside.

I used to love the feeling of everyone looking at me when I was in my Polo, it was so loud they probably thought it was a Ferrari but obviously they were very disappointed. All of my mates had newer cars and I liked to be the odd one out. Before getting my car I upgraded my scooter to an Aprilia SR125 and sold my Italjet to reimburse my Dad. I then did my full bike test and then upgraded my Aprilia to a Gilera Runner VXR 200 (4 stroke). Not as quick as my 2 stroke Aprilia but a smoother ride. My greatest car of all time and quite possibly the greatest car I will ever own was another White Polo MK3 however this was a GT. It was beautiful, I transferred all my sound system from the first one into the new one and bought a new interior of a polo forum I was a member of. I also made a few other minor amendments to the exterior and it was good to go. It had no catalytic convertor on it and a DTM exhaust and it sounded amazing. I used to have to put the cat back on when it needed MOT'ing which was a bit of a mess about. It had a ported and polished head, I don't have a clue what that means but it sounds good. I even had some dice with my name on them which Tina (Tom's Mum) had bought him but I acquired them. It basically looked exactly the same as the CL I had before previously but it so wasn't to a man that knows. I used to wind the sunroof open and wind all the windows down and drive under bridges, the sound it made was like you hear on the F1 footage. I didn't transfer my G2AY T number plate onto this new car for obvious reasons. It did however have German number plates on it, these were actually bought by the previous owner at a show in Wolfsburg, Germany. The rear plate was even White. People used to actually think my car was German, people would ask questions like 'why don't you just drive an English car like everyone else'. I used to get pulled up by the Bobbies all the time and get fined. The GT story unfortunately has a sad end, I sold my car (I took the number plate of the front bumper to keep as a memento and it is hung up on my wall) to my good friend Rob years down the line. Now this is where the story differs between myself and Rob. In my eyes the car was perfect and had nothing wrong with it. Anyway the first day Rob had my car he reversed it onto his drive and crashed it into his living room. He then rings me up to tell me that I have sold him a dodgy car and that upon close inspection is actually 2 cars welded together. Now Rob if you are reading this, my Polo was one car and one car only. You began your life with my car by entering your Mums lounge in it. I'm not sure what happened to it in the end. It was a sad end to a truly amazing car.

My 18th Birthday was quite eventful, we were all out in the Wetherby consuming large amounts of alcohol. The night was great and me and Tom walked into Swallownest for a pizza which was standard practice in those days. I was extremely drunk and can't actually remember what happened but pieced it together from witness accounts. I walked into the chip shop with a sign on my head, this lad asked me to leave but I didn't. Eventually I went outside and all hell went loose. This lad smashed me in my face just above my eye and it split open. Tom was fighting this boxer and had the upper hand, Tom can actually handle himself whereas I can't. In the end the two lads went and I was left with Tom on the street. Tom took me home and my Mum rushed me down to Rotherham General Hospital A&E where it was stitched up. The next day we all went to Skeggy for the night as it was my birthday weekend. I was a little worse for where and was extremely pissed of. We couldn't find a hotel and things were going from bad to worse, I was becoming increasingly angry as I wanted my 18th to be something great that I would remember for the right reasons but it wasn't looking that way. I felt a great deal of failure for myself really, I so badly wanted to be happy with something. We found somewhere and went out, we all went crazy and Skegness had pub watch, most other places didn't have it back then. We all went into Rhino's and ordered a round of drinks, necked them and told the barman we weren't going to pay. The next thing we were all bundled of and that's when they put us on pub watch. I at the time had extremely long hair with a massive gash above my eye, I wasn't exactly Mr Inconspicuous. I lost everyone from that point and didn't know where I was supposed to sleep. Eventually I kipped on a roundabout near the sea front. I woke up that morning rather confused and just as I stood up all the lads were walking down the street. They couldn't believe what they saw before them.

It was around this time when I started going out with my first girlfriend, her name was Lucy. She was great and I guess now looking back on it, she was my first love. We spent a lot of time together and did a lot of things, she was and still is a fantastic girl and I owe her a lot. It was one of the best things I've ever experienced, getting to know each other and doing all the things couples do. We went to Amsterdam and ate some dodgy muffins as well as always going out into the Peak District for meals. We thought we were set up for life.

The problem with having a girlfriend was I fell out of the loop a bit with the lads and I wanted to be one of the lads so much. At first it didn't matter to me that I was missing out on things as I was caught up in this romance but that didn't last unfortunately, in the end after over a year I decided I wanted to be on my own, this was because I felt if I didn't have a girlfriend I could be out with my mates and become really popular. It was around the time just before we finished that I remember feeling very low and looking back possibly unhappy. I felt I wasn't liked, I also felt that people didn't want to be my mate as much as they did with other people. I was 18 at this point and I decided to finish the relationship. For some crazy reason we went to a place called Derwent Valley and it was half way around the lake that I told Lucy I wanted to be on my own, so I then had to walk the rest of the way around the lake (2 hours) and all the way back to Sheffield with this girl who's heart I felt I had just broken. I did it in the kindest way I thought possible although I hated myself for it especially as I knew how much she loved me but I couldn't continue with the relationship as I knew in the long run she would be better of without me as my feelings had changed greatly.

I thought if I was on my own my popularity would soar and I could become this person I had in my head that I wanted to be. In my deluded head I thought it would make me happy and the relationship was the reason for my unhappiness. In reality the ideals I had in my mind where not actually that great but more of a pipedream. In summary Lucy and I had a fantastic year together and you never actually forget your first true love.

4. AFROMAN

In sixth form I didn't have a clue what I wanted to do with the rest of my life except that I wanted to be rich and successful. I didn't put too much time or effort into how I would achieve these ambitions. I set very high standards for myself without any major plan in getting there, unbeknown to me at the time was I was setting myself up for a fall. I decided I wanted to go out and meet lots of different women and 'play the field' a bit, this was a desire that would take me half away around the world. I just wanted to have the best things and be the best at everything, I'm not sure why as I wasn't ever that good at anything. This is in stark contrast to how I was in secondary school, I didn't have such wild fantasies of being rich or successful, I just got on with life and was happy with what I had. Something had changed within me that now meant I needed success to be happy. I've tried to go more back to that way of thinking I had in secondary school and to get out of an unhappy loop I get myself into due to having such high ambitions. It's hard because for such a long time I wanted so badly to be successful at something and I feel like its ingrained into my personality and no matter how much I try it's always there.

One time at sixth form I had a competition with a school friend called Alex, we bet £5 who would have their hair cut first, we said if neither of us has it cut after a year we will call it a draw, now I think he was pulling my plonker as his hair never seemed to grow, I believe he was secretly having it cut without telling me. My mop on the other hand was getting out of control and was extremely curly, once Lucy straightened it and it went down to my shoulders. I think I won the bet! It's hard to explain how big my afro was but it was massive and created much attention. I then went from having it all long to then shaving it all off with a bic razor. I've still got the hair in a bag upstairs with all my hair in, the barbers must have thought I was crackers firstly for going from an afro to bald and secondly collecting my hair in a carrier bag. Later on that day I remember meeting all the lads in Meadowhall with Lucy and they couldn't believe what I had done. That kind of summarised my personality, I was all or nothing, very extreme.

I found sixth form hard at times, I was struggling with the feelings of not been popular enough or not being the person I wanted to be. Those feelings of 'just being' had disappeared and I was back to how I felt in junior school. It's funny when I'm feeling fine I don't have these worries of acceptance but when I get down or am put in stressful situations then these are the feelings that arise. I wouldn't say I get depressed about the feelings in general but it just gets me down. If I don't get out of that cycle then things start to spiral out of control and depression can creep in. I often felt like I wasn't the person I wanted to be and that I wasn't living life to the full and that hurt. I wanted every second of my life to be the best it could be and that in itself is a very tiring way of living but it's what I thought would make me happy.

I did well with my A-Levels, I got an A in Geography, B in Economics and a E in Design Technology. Firstly Geography was the greatest subject to study for me, we had two fantastic teachers, Mr Lyon and Mr Hodgeson. Mr Hodgeson was our sixth form leader and was an extremely interesting and funny man he reminded me of Jeremy Clarkson, Mr Lyon was much more subtle but equally as interesting. I loved every minute of Geography and I learned a lot about the physical and human side of the subject. Plus I found the work pretty easy for a change and was actually good at it. We had a great class and a class that the teachers said was one of the best ones they had taught. It was Proc who came up with my nickname, Trigger. This was based on The Only Fools and Horses character. Proc told me that I too was a bit daft like Trigger. So that name stuck and a few friends still call it me now. We went on some fantastic field trips including the Isle of Arran to study glaciers and York to study the human effects industrialisation, the class was great and we had a few funny characters and a great bunch of girls and we all got on great. The theories within the subject are very transferable. It's strange writing this as it all seems like such happy times but there were times when things weren't so good. I've read many an autobiography and you read it and realise that many people go through tough times and that success wasn't just handed to them on a plate.

Economics was also a magical time and I loved the teacher again as well as the course content. Mr Hadfield was a fantastic teacher and he made the course extremely interesting plus Mr Long also was a very knowledgeable man. From there it goes downhill mainly as I was reunited with my good friend Tom again. Lucy was in my class and we hadn't started going out at this point in time so my mind wasn't exactly on the job. My main goal from that class was getting with Lucy and having a laugh with Tom. These were 2 goals I achieved but unfortunately at the price of getting a good grade. We had a good time in those Design Tech days, I made a trolley for my final project and Tom made a bike stand. Both were equally as crap and our written project work was equally as shocking. My other old junior school friend Richard started the course but didn't finish it as he left to pursue a career in golf. He would later turn out to be a very good friend indeed. He went missing after leaving sixth form, not actually missing but he went off the scene for a while just as we started going out drinking and he made some good mates at golf and managed to get his handicap down to plus 1 which if you have ever played golf will appreciate what an achievement this is.

Me and Tom bought ourselves an X-Plorer pit bike each, these were basically 4 stroke off road motorbikes but with very small frames, we looked like a right set of plonkers on them. It was so good to go out exploring and going to all these interesting areas nearby, there were so many places to see. It was something I wanted to do from an early age but was never able to get a bike so here I was at 17 living out my childhood dream. We went all over and we went to new places all the time, they were so small we could get over any obstacles in our way and over any of the barriers aimed at stopping bikes. Sometimes we would ride to Chesterfield all of road on the Trans Pennine Trail, this of course wasn't strictly legal but we had to ride them somewhere. On this one occasion we were riding for a while up near an area called Spinkhill and we came across this tunnel, it was all over grown and dark and we ventured in. It turned out it was in passable and we had to turn around but it was incredibly eerie and reminded me of something from Lost. After a while Kidder bought himself a bike and he was a fantastic rider and he too joined the gang, finally Richard and Ben also purchased bikes and Richard had a van so we could venture further a field. On one occasion we went into Sherwood Forrest in Nottingham and rid around there for ages it was so much fun, then of course the local fuzz had to turn up and spoil our day and give us a section 22 each! Once we went all the way to a quarry in Doncaster and I rode my bike straight into a ditch and snapped my rear wheel so we all went home! Think I lasted 10 minutes.

5.   THE ENTERTAINER

It was in those early days at sixth form that I discovered alcohol and this really fuelled my problems. I was trying so hard to be somebody that I wasn't that I failed to appreciate what I had got. I would go out with the sole intention of getting hammered, not just to go and have a sociable couple of drinks but to get paralytic. I would always try to be the centre of attention and I loved the attention I would get from it. It was as if I turned into somebody else. I would get high and at the time I thought everyone loved it too. Maybe they were maybe they weren't I'm not too sure. What I do know is I turned into the person I always wanted to be and that was the entertainer. We drank a lot, there was always an 18th birthday party at the Swallownest Social Club and I used to drink Stones and it was so cheap as the social club wasn't part of a brewery. A lot of the time I could handle the hangovers as it was the price I had to pay to be the man I wanted to be. It's just so sad that I couldn't without a drink. It was around this age that I became obsessed with fire extinguishers and for sale signs. Someone would always wake up Sunday morning and realise their house was now on the market. Every weekend would involve the redistribution of a for sale sign. On one occasion some poor unsuspecting drive-thru attendant became the poor victim of the fire extinguisher attack. Once we actually locked the whole staff in McDonalds inside by slotting a piece of wood in the door which meant they were stuck, we just stood outside laughing. Things like this happened on a weekly basis and the fun we had was something special and unique.

But very often I wouldn't get high after drinking but I'd get low and when the drink failed to make me popular or the man of the moment, I would then go into decline and it could last for days after the event. I used to buzz off everyone talking about me and telling stories that were about me, I craved that attention and external acceptance. It was just a shame I was a boring twat when I was sober. Sometime before I had even had a drink I would be buzzing in the house as I knew I was going out and I knew I was going to put on a wicked show for everyone. Just the thought of it made me happy. But that external gratification wasn't always there and when it wasn't I'd do even more stupid things to try and get it. A lot of people thought I was a complete dick and I can't for one minute blame them, when drunk I was and would probably be the same now after 10 pints. I wasn't alone in this drunken behaviour I had my wing man Tom. He was a character as well and on good days we'd both buzz off each other. We'd get in the occasional bit of bother but Tom could handle himself and I couldn't fight myself out of a paper bag. We used to go down Rotherham in our Stone Island jumpers and we thought we were football hooligans, I even read a book about the BBC (Blades Business Crew as apposed to the television people). We used to end up getting in scuffles, once this lad messed Anthony's hair up, so Ant told Tom and he confronted this lad, the next thing this other lad comes out of nowhere and lands on right on my nose, blood started pouring out so I ran in the toilet. I was in a right mess I was crying my eyes out and sobbing saying its all your fault Tom you cause all this trouble. What a big girls blouse I was. I ended up attempting to walk home but it was freezing so I walked back into town and got a taxi. Once Sam decided to jump on a lorry that stopped in the traffic outside the club, he then went for miles on the back of this lorry and had to get a taxi back.

I should have seen the alarm bells - once on this trip we all went to Amsterdam, we were on this boat travelling overnight. I drank a large quantity of Gin (as I felt shocking mentally on the trip, totally out of place) and became extremely depressed and found myself on the top floor of the boat thinking about jumping off. On the boat it felt like everybody was having fun and I just felt all alone. The only way I knew how to deal with this was to drink, and drink a lot. The next day I just put it down to just being drunk. We continued with our weekend trip and my mood wasn't as low however there were some of the early signs that I had problems.

I decided I wanted to do Economics at University, this was mainly down to my Economic teacher at Sixth Form, as already discussed he was a legend. He used to tell us all about stories from his youth and made a really good connection with the students. He also studied Economics, so I thought if I study economics then I'll turn out like my teacher - talk about being naive. I managed to get a B in Economics at A level, I worked very hard for that and I think the result was also down to some top quality teaching, I even got full marks on one paper. I decided on a bit of a whim that I would go to Nottingham Trent University, a fellow student Hussain told me that the nightlife in Nottingham was very good. I didn't even go round the University or the Halls or even read a prospectus, one of the deciding factors was I was under the impression that there was a ratio of men to women of 1 in 5 in Nottingham. Now I don't think that was true at the time, maybe at one time this might have been the case but it certainly wasn't when I got there. I probably should have chosen a different course as there were not many girls on the course! It was around the start of University that I decided I wanted to spread my wings and I thought with the 1 in 5 ratio I'd probably meet loads more women, how wrong could I be. As I mentioned Lucy and I split up around the start of University, Lucy took my decision reasonably well I felt, I heard from other people that she was a little upset but this was understandable, we had a very good relationship and it was a shame it had to finish. I think I was depressed at the time, not majorly but I was a lost soul at that point in my life and I thought if I was single then I would get to where I wanted to go. Lucy was a fantastic first girlfriend and I had a smashing time, she is now settled down with a boyfriend, we don't speak a lot but I often wonder how she is.

So here I was in a new city, at a new University and a new start. I think my problems first began when I started drinking but increased more around the time I left for University. I used to drink then and up until recently far too much, I used to drink until I couldn't drink anymore and it was mainly Vodka. But from drinking was borne a new personality: Drunk Tom. I remember one of the only few girls on the course Rose saying to me 'you're so funny when your drunk' and this made me feel like I needed to be drunk in order to gain popularity or be entertaining. And this is what I did, I just drank so that I could be 'funny'. I failed to look at how destructive this could be. Looking back I can see strong links between my illness and my late teens and early twenties, my mood used to go sky high when I was drinking and then I would have the inevitable down period, this was like a hangover but much worse. Sometimes I would come out with the conclusion that I was a waste of space and worthless. I remember at University having suicidal thoughts. This was because I thought all my problems would disappear once I got to University but in truth they just followed me. Plus there was the added problem of not being around any of my friends and family to contend with. I lived away from home Monday to Thursday and came home to work Fridays and Saturdays at the petrol station. Even though I wasn't away a great deal I still felt like I was missing out on things at home with my pals and family. Looking back on the start of university it was a very tough time, I made the decision to leave Lucy and start University for all the wrong reasons and it had back fired on me. I remember my family coming to see me in Nottingham and we all went out for tea, I was really low and didn't have any appetite. I didn't know why I wasn't eating but looking back now I know it was because I was depressed. Before going to University it gave me hope that my life would change for the better. I believed that my whole personality would be transformed and I would become this really talkative, funny popular kid. This of course didn't happen and I withdrew even further.

During my time at Nottingham Trent I did try the odd bit of Marijuana but it didn't do anything for me, it made me feel really tired and I always felt ill. I wanted to be high as in buzzing. It was around then when I started out at University that I had my first experience of trying Ecstasy. Now that was more for me and it agreed with my body more. The first time I tried it was on a night out in Sheffield when I was with my mates from home, it was a really powerful and amazing experience. All these chemicals were rushing around my head, all of my problems were gone and I just felt this overwhelming feeling of love for everyone and everything. I didn't need to talk to people I just got in your own zone and listened to the music, I found peace within yourself. For me who was at war with myself this was incredible. I hate to talk about the positive side of drug abuse but I understand why people take the drug. A few months later we all went to a trance night called Gatecrasher which was held at an old steel works called Magna near Meadowhall. I remember whilst under the influence of the drug saying to a girl in Gatecrasher "imagine if every day of your life was like this". I used to love going to Gatecrasher, the music was great and the atmosphere was amazing. I had such a good time at these events it was untrue, I think it was mainly down to the music. There was an abundance of ecstasy at these events, I remember having 2 pills but nothing happened, then some more. Nothing was happening so I took 3 more. I took so many its untrue, I'm not even going to say how many as you probably won't believe me. Anyway all of a sudden I felt this tidal wave of immense good feeling rush through me and they kicked in. Well I've never known anything like it, I must have shook hands with 90% of the people in the club. When I was walking it felt I was on one of those moving walkways you get at the airport. My body was gliding through the clouds but my feet weren't moving. When I did actually move my legs and walk I just moved even faster past everyone, it was just like walking on air. I was on top, my doubts in life where long gone. I was in the moment, me, the music and the people. We came out of the club around 6am and I was in no state to go home so I got the mini bus driver to take me into town. From there I just walked around until I came down a little. Then of course the payment plan sinks in. The days after taking the drug are awful, it almost sends you into a depressed state. But it's like most things in life, everything has a price and you have to weigh it up. I only tried it a few times and luckily for me I didn't get hooked on the stuff. Some people chase that high and it can sometimes lead to more problems down the line. I've been to Ibiza a few times and there is a big drug problem over there but where there is a party there will always be drugs.

I met a great friend at University called Francis, I remember the first night with all the people from the Halls, me and Francis just bonded really well and it ended up me and him being out on our own until the early hours, he had a Paul and Shark jumper on which I thought was rare for a student. I too had a Paul and Shark t-shirt on, sounds daft but little things like that can say a lot about a person. Once I got to know him it turned out we were very similar and had a similar past with regards larking about with our mates. We had a lot of fun. I remember one night coming back to our Halls and we decided to smash the kitchen to pieces, I haven't a clue why, but the next morning was deadly. The other residents thought we had been burgled, there were eggs scattered about the place, frying pans were in the garden, the lot went. So Francis and I had an amazing time, I don't think I would have lasted my first year without him. It was just like going out with one of my mates from back home. By now all I wanted to do was go out drinking, my passion for Economics had diminished somewhat but I still tried hard with my studies. I got 56% in my first year which wasn't bad given the fact that I was struggling with my own issues and I was constantly drunk. There were some interesting people on my course but I didn't make much effort in getting to know them, I still lacked massively in confidence in groups. I just came to the conclusion that people aren't interested in me and it comes back to that whole issue of not feeling good enough about myself. If I can't entertain the group to my high standards then I think why bother. It's a very destructive cycle as I then beat myself up for not trying. Whilst I was feeling very down in myself and somewhat lost with the world my old junior school friends decided to have a school reunion at a pub in the village and as well as everyone else Tom and Richard went along for the event one Thursday night. However nobody decided to invite me, not even my supposedly close friends and once I found out everyone went along to the party without me I felt crushed, it was as if I didn't exist. I felt so alone in the world around this point and had come to the conclusion that I was not wanted and by my close friends not even having the audacity to invite me to the reunion just reaffirmed what I already felt. They had given me evidence to support my theory.

There is only one thing in life worse than being talked about, and that is not being talked about.

The main aim of my move to Nottingham was to become a different person, to re-invent myself but now I know it's not possible to have a personality change, but that is exactly what I wanted, I would drink, take or do anything to try and achieve my goal of becoming more liked and more respected. There was another lad who I knew from back home called Adam, he was an old family friend and we used to play golf together in the early days. I met up with Adam on a number of occasions he was really funny but I really struggled to fit in with him and his mates, I just couldn't seem to feel happiness or contentment. We would all go out but I believed that nobody wanted to be around me, there is perhaps some truth attached to that. The last time I saw Adam was in Oceana which was a big nightclub in Nottingham. He was sat in this area with a girl he was seeing at the time, I was with Tom at the time and we were on one right that night. Anyway I saw him and decided to go and pick up a bucket full of ice and chuck in over the pair of them. I don't have a clue why but I did it. This might possibly be the first ever Ice Bucket Challenge. Like many things I have done in my life I fail to see reasoning behind my actions. Such acts lead me further away from my need to feel more liked and respected. Rightly so Adam has never had a great deal to do with me since.

On a separate occasion when Tom came to see me, we had a few drinks in the halls, in fact we played centurion with Kronenburg and lasted about 30 minutes. If you don't know what that is you simply have a shot of beer every minute for 100 minutes, it sounds easy but it is very difficult but it gets you plastered and serves a purpose. We left my halls and entered the grassy area in the middle off all the halls. There was a group of lads so we headed over to them, something happened and we ended up getting chased by a group of about 10 lads who were congregated outside. I'm not sure what happened but one of the lads tried throwing a car battery at us. We legged it and hid in some gardens down the road for what seemed like ages.

Eventually we got to town and as per usual we thought we ran the city. We headed into the lace market and went to some fancy bars and we were having the time of our lives. It was pre smoking ban so we were both sat in Tantra's with big fat Cuban cigars drinking Southern Comfort and Lemonade. The bill Tom had for 2 drinks and 2 cigars was £34, he still has the card receipt. I'm not sure why we had this sense of power, almost like we were better than everyone else but back then we did. Prior to Tantra's we went to Pizza Hut and I'm pretty ashamed now I'm older about what happened but hey ho. We went into Pizza Hut and ordered 2 Stella's and looked at the menu. We then ordered our meal and some more Stella. We waited a while and got our pizza and demolished it. We then decided that it would be a good idea to eat our pizzas, drink up and fuck of. We smashed back our last glass and made our exit. We casually walked out of the restaurant, hearts beating ten to the dozen and legged it once we were in the street. I followed Tom. He ran about 200 yards and hid behind a Biffa bin. Of all the places in Nottingham to run too he picks a bin next to the restaurant. So we were stuck there for ages and didn't know where to go. Eventually we got out and didn't get caught. I've since been to pizza hut and paid something like £20 for a pizza. How can a student be expected to eat paying those prices. After Tantra's we got in some other bother with a student from Trent, I'm not sure why there was an altercation but all I can remember is Tom trying to ram a traffic barrier through this kids flat front door. It looked like something from a medieval film where they go through the castle front door with a tree trunk. This lad was shitting it and he was throwing eggs at us. We just stood at the bottom laughing. Eventually we had to leave the scene and just as we left the area and police car turned up. Not tonight Mr Policeman, you'll need a special sat nav to catch Tom Tom.

I lost Tom later on that night and was on my own. I was it a real mess and couldn't walk very well due to the copious amounts of drinks we had consumed. I managed to flag a taxi driver down and I got in. I didn't have any cash but did have my bank card. So we stopped at a cash machine on the way home. I got out of the taxi and went up to the cash machine and put my card in. I tried to enter my pin number but couldn't focus on the key pad and kept pressing the wrong numbers. So I asked the taxi driver if he would do it for me and I gave him my card and told him my pin number. He then ran into his car and drove of with my card and pin. I was then stuck with nothing. How stupid can you get? He withdrew £450 out. Well given the events prior to that I deserved some kind of punishment.

'Do unto others as you would have others do unto you'.

During sixth form everyone thought I looked like Mike Skinner from the Streets and he soon became my idol. I used to wear the same clothes and always listen to his music. I thought if I did everything he did I'd turn into the type of person he was. His songs were like instructions on how to live your life. What I failed to realise was even if I became the next Mike Skinner I still wouldn't be happy. One of his lyrics is "ran from a cab like a mad little lout" so I thought I'd have to do that. The problem was when we tried it my mate got his coat stuck in the door so we had to pay. But still it was another thing off the Skinner's 'to do' list. If you ever listen to his songs they have a strong theme running through them, and that's drugs, maybe that was why I was fascinated in trying different types of drugs. I guess I just craved that admiration he had from a large amount of people, I naively believed that becoming that sort of person would lead me to happiness. What it did was drove me in the opposite direction, I was heading in the complete opposite path of where I wanted to be however I didn't have a clue how I could change course. All I kept doing was repeating the same behaviour and that was drinking to extremes.

We went to see the Streets at Plug in Sheffield, I went along with my Aquascutum checked long sleeve shirt and my Stone Island hoody. I tried my best to look like him, the night was great and we went to a VIP room where he was DJ'ing. As I went in there was a big group of girls so I went over and introduced myself as Tom Skinner the brother of Mike. These chicks were buying this and it went on for sometime. Then Beat Stevie came over and wanted to interview me. So I did and even made up a little wrap for them. It was a poor attempt admittedly. On a separate occasion I was in a bar in Nottingham and I started talking to this girl at the bar, I told her I was Mike Skinner and she just grabbed me and started kissing me.

On one of my many visits home I was sat watching Lost on the PC in the spare bedroom. I was just into my second bottle of rose when my phone rang. It was my friend Chad, he said he'd got us a crazy party organised and there was an abundance of birds for us. So I agreed to go and he picked me up in his Suzuki Swift. We headed of to Barnsley and I continued to drink my nice bottle of Black Tower. We ended up in the town centre and we were lost and didn't know where this place was where we were supposed to be going. So Chad decides it's a good idea to ask two policeman who were on the road next to us at the lights. Bearing in mind he didn't have a licence, tax or insurance. The car had an MOT so it wasn't so bad. The police said, 'were not sure but those lads behind will know'. So we looked behind us and it was a paddy wagon full of them. They must have done a check on the car. So Chad puts it in first and wheel spins it up a one way street and the van followed us closely in pursuit with the lights and sirens. We drove around Barnsley for a bit and we thought we had lost them, he pulled into a car park and jumps over this wall and onto a roof. I tried to climb up the wall but couldn't get up, I had no strength. I told Chad to run but he didn't. By this point all the police ran towards us, we were in a corner and we had been captured. We were put in the van and sent to Barnsley police station. I was very drunk by now and was shouting at all these police officers accusing them of abuse and a whole host of other things. I told them I had taken drugs and if they didn't let me leave I'd take some more. This resulted in me having to wait for a doctor for an assessment. They let us out in the early morning once I had sobered up. Chad is one of the most loyal people I know, he's extremely tough on the outside but has a great heart. Bit like a Rolo. He later joined the Marines however discharged on the grounds of ill health. If things were different for him growing up I'm sure he could have made a career as a professional boxer. His passion however is dogs now and he has an exceptional connection with them.

The course was going well, but I just wasn't happy there. The Halls of Residence I was staying at were the worst out of the lot, this was because I had left it so late to apply. My room was basically like a prison cell, it wasn't even plastered just painted breeze blocks. There was a sink in the room with a bed and a desk. We shared all the showers and toilets and also the kitchen. In our block there was a massive variety of people but I never got to know the people very well. I would always shy away from conversation and tended to stay in my room. I spent a lot of time with Francis and we even played cricket down the corridor. As usual we used to get carried away, we used to hit the ball as hard as we could and one time we ended up smashing one of the roof tiles. So we had to go on a little mission to another block and exchange the damaged item. I of course found this very amusing a chuckled though out the whole operation. I had to cycle to the University or catch a bus, this usually took 20 minutes or so and I guess was a good bit of fitness. We didn't have any pubs in walking distance which was a shame, this meant we could never just call for a few pints and wander home.

We did some very interesting parts in the course and I enjoyed all the different modules, the maths teacher Phil was also a bit of a legend. He taught so many useful Mathematical theories that are very useful. He was a fantastic lecturer and dressed more like a student often sporting his Mickey Mouse t shirt. The subjects where very practical and related to the real world, in Economics there are two main parts Macro and Micro, macro talks about the economy as a whole and goes into theories of how certain events can effect economies as a whole and the role the government plays. There are a lot of diagrams and of course not forgetting the very important supply and demand graph. Macro economics become very important after the 2008 crash as it showed how the lending of banks in relation to sub prime mortgages lead to a world wide crisis effecting most of the Western world. Micro economics on the other hand is about individual industries i.e. the oil industry. It also talks about the links between certain industries and how prices are determined. Out of the 2 I preferred Macro as I found it more interesting as it was more relevant. In addition to that we also studied the history of economics, one important topic I was lectured about was the German Hyperinflation in the 20s where inflation was 300% in one month which I found very fascinating, apparently the Germans were pushing wheel barrows around full of cash. We also studied politics and statistics. The course wasn't easy by any means and I did put in a lot of work behind the scenes and when I got too it I found the work very rewarding. Sometimes I would get stuck and I'd try and get the lads on the course to give me a hand but that was difficult as I didn't really socialise with them outside the lectures. So on the whole the course covered a wide range of subjects which were interesting and informative. It's such a shame that my head wasn't in the right place as it was such a great opportunity to grow as a person and get a good qualification behind me and in theory get set up for a good career. But my motives behind university were not to develop as a student but instead transform into a new person. If I could have the head I have now on my 19 year old body then the outcome of University may have been very different. Of course I am only surmising. My demons were never far away, I always had it in my head that people didn't want to sit with me in lectures, I also thought there was a bit of a click and I wasn't in it. The lads on the course were lovely people but just not like my sort of crowd, I'd always just ask random questions to make small talk and never had a laugh. I withdrew myself a bit and tended just to go out with Francis and left the lads on the course too it. I don't know how I'd approach things now if I had the chance. Maybe I'd be kinder to myself, the people who have helped me with my mental health problems have all told me to do that and not set such high standards. For example now I would tell myself that maybe I'm not the class joker or the lad who everyone wants to hang with but in fact I am a decent bloke who maybe isn't meant to be the centre of attention. Maybe I would have found peace within myself and just enjoyed having the small talk and got on with the course. I kind of made the assumption on day one that Uni wasn't for me and that I wasn't going to enjoy it. I never even gave myself the opportunity to discover what may happen. My guard was up from the start.

6. FIREMAN SAM

On this one occasion Tom came down to see me at Nottingham for one reason or another and we decided we would go out on the town, for some reason we decided we would take the polo down to Loughborough University as we had heard it was a good place to go and we knew Sally who was a resident there. So we set of down to Loughborough. Anyway we gets a call that Sam and Chad were going to be there, so we all met up. The night started of ok and we got a few drinks down us then I bumped into an old junior school friend Richard (not my mate Richard) anyway this person wasn't a friend at all and in all fairness was a complete dick with me that night and we ended up scrapping, nothing serious. I think he has a few hang ups from back in the day and something I did or said still bothers him but it just showed to me how much of a waster he actually is. So there was this little skirmish in the union. That's that and we continued drinking, we were drinking snake bites and they were going back like nobody's business. There was a dance group on the union stage which comprised of students. They were all on the stage doing a routine in front of the crowd. I thought it was a good idea to pull my hood up and go dancing with all the girls. I was having a great time and looked like some sort of grim reaper come Michael Jackson act. This was until I was carried off by the bouncers. So from there I was physically exited and told I wouldn't be going back in and they gave me a lifetime ban from Loughborough University Student Union. I'm not sure how they are going to police the lifetime ban, one day I'm going to go back to see if they recognise me. So we were all now stuck outside the union and we didn't know what to do with ourselves and in the distance were two towers and one of us just pointed and said lets go there. So we headed off to these two towers that were in the distance all unsure what would meet us there upon our arrival. When we got there we jumped in the lift and went straight to the top. We got out of the lift and we were greeted by a collection of fire extinguishers. No words were spoken, it was just a natural thing to do. We all armed ourselves with a fire extinguisher each then we made our way down to the next level and knocked on all the doors of all the rooms like some sort of terrorist raid, as soon as someone answered the door we all sprayed them with our fire extinguishers and then ran off, we repeated this until we ran out of water. Then some bright spark decided to upgrade his weapon to the big hose and proceeded to saturate any poor sole that was unfortunate enough to open their door. That must be where they get the name from for the TV show.....Fireman Sam.

By the time we reached the bottom the lift opened up and there stood about 10 security guards, they were blocking all the exits. We all looked at each other and were all formulating a plan in our heads. I froze, I didn't know what to do. Chad and Sam made a B line for the fire exit. The security guards where stood there but soon moved. If you knew Chad and Sam you would let them out, the door was kicked straight off its hinges. This just left me and Tom, we waited for about 10 minutes and the security guards weren't sure what to do with us. Anyway after a while the local Bobbies arrived. Two officers came up to us and me and Tom just looked at each other and then in unison put our wrists out and then we were arrested. We were taken down to Loughborough Police Station and put in cells. I knew I was in trouble as I had all the plastic security tags from the extinguishers and I believed they would use these as evidence against me. We were put in our cells and we stayed there for some time. Tom told me after that they gave him magazines and made him a meal but they never did that for me! Not sure why as I was very compliant, I had learnt that from my last stint in the slammer. Anyway they rang a solicitor for me and I spoke with this guy on the phone, I believed they would simply just listen to the call and hear my story. Bit of paranoia there for you. Once we had sobered up they interviewed us, it turned out that Sam and Chad got caught in the end in Chad's car making a getaway from the campus, they were also being questioned at the police station. Chad was sent down South to be questioned by the Marine Police for a separate issue. So I made my statement and basically just said it was a drunken prank that got out of hand and that we didn't mean any harm by it, this was the truth. It was a little frightening really as you can't speak to your mates to find out what they are going to say and get your facts in line. The cells were, as all cells, cold and dark with a dirty blanket. I managed to sleep for a while and then I just lay there mulling over things in my mind. I suppose I knew we'd be let out as it wasn't anything serious but doubt always creeps into your mind. I did however know one thing, I felt like I was alive, not just subscribing to the bullshit system of watching TV and playing on computer games. I was creating real life drama with my best mates in a way that was immensely entertaining and exciting but causing little damage to people. I mean maybe there have been a few causalities along the way and a few innocent civilians have become soaking wet by a set of amateur fireman but c'mon I've been on the receiving end of a few pranks and what goes around in this world comes around. It's a dog eat dog world out there.

It was just a waiting game until we would found out our fate. I was released with a fine and was informed that there would be no criminal record. When we were finally released we walked out and it was snowing. It was a nice feeling to get our freedom back after my 1 night's incarceration at her majesty's pleasure. We all had a good laugh on the way back up the M1 after that night, there were stories flying everywhere.

I decided after completing year 1 at Nottingham Trent that I would be happier moving to Sheffield as I believed my unhappiness was down to the fact I was not around my friends back home. Again I was just making bad decision after bad decision with the belief that I could find some serenity with myself and just enjoy what was around me.

From being a child we had always driven past the old Sheffield University building, the building is called Firth Court and is a fantastic looking building with ivy growing over the red bricks. From a young age I always wanted to go there so it was a fantastic experience to walk in the building for the first time to get registered, I came out proud as punch and thought this time it will work out this time things will be different. To be accepted at the University of Sheffield is a massive achievement by anybody's standards.

I applied to join a course in Economics to start in the 2nd year at The University of Sheffield and I got accepted, so for the time being this was great. After being accepted I found out I could enter the modules that would change my degree from a BA to a Bsc. This seemed like a no brainer at the time as all I would have to do was enter into the Maths and Econometrics modules. The maths teacher said ideally you need a Maths A Level to enter for the Maths Module but he said in this case he would let me on the course. The content in both the Maths and Econometrics were way above me, it was like I had been entered into the wrong course and in fact I was being taught in Russian. I just did not get the maths and econometrics at all and even went to see a specialist Maths tutor. He looked at my papers and couldn't even do it. Now what chance did I have? He still charged me for informing me of his inadequacies. To make matters worse I didn't speak to one person on the course, I couldn't think of anything to say to any of the students. I couldn't ask them all the normal questions you ask when you're new as I felt they would have answered them all in the first year. Like where are you from? Where are you staying? What's your view on the current interest rates? Are you single? That kind of thing. So I said nothing. It was such an overwhelmingly lonely time worse so than Nottingham. When I'm unhappy I just make plans to do something as I believe it is the situation or environment that I am in that is the problem. The truth is the problem is deep within my sole and has little to do with any other external factors. My confidence was practically none existence and I literally did not speak to one person for my entire time at Sheffield. This wonderful world was all around me but I couldn't grasp it.

You are probably recognising a repeat from Nottingham Trent, well it was. I would struggle somewhere i.e. at home, then move to somewhere totally new i.e. Nottingham. I then find my problems have followed me so I try to start afresh i.e. The University of Sheffield. This happened throughout my childhood with sport or the air cadets for example. I literally repeated the same cycle over and over again and never made any progress. Would I ever stop doing this?

It was around this time when I went down town with a couple of friends and we stopped by at a shop on West Street that sold 'legal highs' so I bought quite a few and I also drank copious amounts of alcohol and we ended up in the Republic Nightclub. I lost everyone and was in a real mess, I don't know if it was the alcohol or the legal highs. Anyway I came out of the nightclub and saw a girl I knew called Holly who was sat with her friend Clare, she jokingly said I'm going to ring your Mum about being drunk. A switch flicked in my brain and I lost all control of my emotions. I ran down the street kicking all the taxi's that were parked along the road. Once I got to the end of the taxi queue I kept running, just outside the nightclub entry was another taxi parked up. I just kept running and ran up the boot of the car, onto the rear windscreen which fell through, then on the roof and down the bonnet making a complete mess of the bodywork putting dints everywhere. I then just carried on running by which point the police were following me in pursuit. My TAG watch broke when I landed on the ground and fell of so I decided to stop and get it. I then set of running again but the police grabbed me and subsequently arrested me. You hear horror stories about these legal highs and to be fair in my experience they are lethal. It was just crazy what I did, to cause that much damage in such a short amount of time was horrifying. They cuffed me up and held me for a while just next to the club. There were quite a few coppers surrounding me. Unlike the fire extinguisher incident this time I was frightened. Once it was all over I sobered up due to the amount of adrenaline that was flowing around my body. I couldn't understand what had happened, what will my parents say as of course Holly had witnessed the whole event along with half of Sheffield. At that moment in my life when I was handcuffed outside the club I knew my head was messed up and needed help. All the negatives where rushing through my head about Uni and who I was as a person. I just did not have a clue what to do next or who to turn to. I couldn't put my finger on what was wrong with me, I couldn't go and see someone and say this is wrong with me or that. It was a universal mess that was beyond outside help. It just so happened that all the cells were full that night both in Sheffield and Doncaster so they would not be taking me into the police station. I made an agreement to pay for the damage and the taxi driver kindly said I would only have to pay the excess and not for the whole windscreen and the damage to the rest of the car.

I made contact with the taxi driver a few days later and agreed to go and pay him. I was very nervous about the meeting but told myself I got myself into the trouble and I therefore would have to get out of it myself. We arranged to meet at the Grosvenor Hotel in Sheffield. I was there on time, the taxi driver pulled up and wound down his window, there were two of them. He seemed like a nice guy and told me to get in the car, I said why do I need to get in, he just said we need to go and get the receipt. I said I don't want a receipt and he just said get in the car, we started to argue a bit. I then decided I had to get out of here, I was extremely frightened now. I thought why on earth do they want me in their car? What are they going to do to me? The next thing I remember was running through the hotel underground car park, I didn't have a clue where I was running too but I was just running. For some reason I decided to run to West Bar police station, I saw a policeman getting into a police car and I stopped him. I told him the circumstances but he sent me on my way saying it wasn't his problem. Now I was even more frightened. I was just panicking and just pacing around the streets thinking every car that went past or stopped was them. I knew that if they found me I was in trouble. I rang Tom and he said he would come into town and meet me. I planned with Tom that I should meet the taxi drivers in the train station, this way it was busier and they would be less likely to drag me into the car. On the night when I actually ran up the taxi the taxi driver agreed he would only want the excess, looking back on it now I think they were just saying that so I would turn up. So I met them in the heavily populated train station, I made sure I was on the CCTV and handed over my £60. The window on the taxi that I smashed was massive and it would have cost a good few hundred pounds plus of course all the bodywork was dented this again made me feel they had other plans for me! Who knows what might have happened to me if I had got in the car. Truth is I probably deserved it.

On the night I ran up the taxi I had no money or wallet and couldn't get home, I never took a bank card out as I would always spend more money than I could afford or buy people drinks, I had also stopped taking my phone out with me as I always used to ring people up when I was drunk, usually to tell them I loved them but at 3am it probably wasn't convenient. The next day I would be extremely embarrassed. So here I was, alone, walking up the middle of the parkway which is the main artery out of Sheffield, it was freezing and there was frost on the ground. All I had one was a thin top, I have never felt cold like it before or since my teeth were chattering and my bones were aching. The walk home is about 10 miles and of the top of my head takes 4 hours the temperature was below zero. I pulled my arms out of my sleeves and crossed them under my top to try and keep the warmth in. I just kept walking, the only thought I had was my bed. The thought of getting out of the cold and into my bed was the single thing that kept me going. I made a decision whilst walking alone up the parkway, I decided I needed to get away, I yet again thought by doing so it would make me a happier person. I think I knew things weren't right, I was struggling with the course at Sheffield and I had no friends on the course to help me or even give me company. I felt very alone and isolated once more. My attitude was all wrong and I wasn't finding life very easy at the time and as always was turning to the drink on an ever increasing scale. Anyway I decided in what seems like an instance that I would leave Sheffield and head to Australia as I couldn't cope with life as it was. But of course as we have already discussed the problems follow you. At this point I owed about £7,000 in University loans for which I did not have a single thing to show for it except and shed load of memories most of which were bad ones. Don't get me wrong it wasn't all bad and I firmly believe life sometimes chooses our path, at the time it feels shit and you ask yourself why me yet there comes a point and you look back and realise 'yes, I now know why that happened because if that didn't happen then I wouldn't be where I am today'. Sometimes it takes you a quarter of a century to discover that, more often than not it takes much longer but eventually you realise. Not an easy thought to posses when everything in your life is going in the complete opposite direction to where you want it to go. But it all makes sense one day.

The New Year that followed the taxi incident was quite an eventful one. Tom and I went round all of the pubs drinking and we had a lot to drink and we were extremely drunk. We ended up in the Yellow Lion and had New Year in there which was great. The next events are very blurred for everyone included, but we ended up walking into another pub called the Blue Bell. In there were another group of lads who Tom was having a bit of trouble with. As I was good mates with Tom I got dragged into all the trouble. The lad who Tom was having all this trouble with even took it upon himself to throw a brick at my car earlier on in the year and made a right mess of it resulting in a costly repair bill. At the time he vandalised my car he didn't have anything against me, in fact he was very close friends with Chris across the road and even used to stand and talk to me so Christ knows why he felt he could take out his frustrations on life against my car. He never actually apologised for this act nor reimbursed me for the expense incurred for painting the roof. Anyway they were all in the Bell. We walked in and it was very controversial what happened next, some say we went it to start a fight and others say we didn't but like I say no one will ever know the truth. What ended up happening were about six lads who were a good 6 years older than us and a grown man who was my Dads age ended up giving Tom an horrendous beating. He ended up losing his front tooth and injuring his cheekbone and was very badly injured. He was in a right mess and I mean a right mess. Some people never recover mentally from such a hiding but what these lads fail to know is Tom's a tough kid, I don't mean he could smash them all up if it was one on one but I mean mentally. I can't imagine what it's like for 6 thugs to set about you. The fear must be horrifying. But it just goes to show what type of people were dealing with. They weren't after me. They did little harm to me apart from grab me and hold me in that jennel across from the pub and make me watch my mate get savagely beaten. I came away with very few injuries that night but what I came away with was guilt. I watched Tom get seriously injured, beaten black and blue and did nothing about it, my oldest friend was lying on the floor in a pool of blood while they were kicking him in his head. And all I did was watch. I wanted my face kicking in, I wanted to be hurt that way I could feel I did something but I had nothing. My failure to Tom that night still haunts me. Although I'm sure Tom doesn't think this but I often wonder does he think I didn't try to help? Does he think I just stood there? I ask myself what did I do to help? Not enough is the answer not enough. The weeks following Tom had serious injuries on his face and the damage they had inflicted was obvious. He didn't look good. I had nothing, not even a scratch. I think deep down I know I did all I could but I can't even be kind enough to myself to believe that, I have the faintest of memories of just screaming at them to stop but they just carried on beating. That night changed me and Tom. Tom for obvious reasons more, I'm not sure in what way but you can't go through that torture and not become reprogrammed in some way. I just became more lost, I'm a very loyal person and at that time in my life Tom was like a brother and I had massively let him down. I can deal with fucking up at Uni but not preventing such torment to my friend hurt deep down. I don't think I realised at the time how much those nights events affected my underlying subconscious. I'm not sure how but it just added into my overwhelming feeling of uselessness. No one ever said anything to me or not to my face anyway but people talk behind your back. Tom never pressed charges against the 6 men in question and they still go about there daily business in and around the village. Now I'm older I feel these people should have been brought to justice for what they did that night. I wonder if they ever feel any remorse for what they did to my pal Tom? Unfortunately I don't think they do.

7. WALKABOUT

I hastily booked flights to Australia and as usual made very few plans and didn't have any realistic visions of what actually might present itself when I got there. All I thought was everything will be alright in Oz.

I can't even remember why I wanted to go to Australia; I didn't exactly think about it too much, I just wanted to get away. It was just my life as a whole I think, I was getting further and further away from living any sort of life that I wanted too. I'm not sure how much longer I stayed at University for after the taxi incident, it was weeks and not months. There was however enough time to get my results from one of my Econometrics exams and that was 18%! I booked my flight, I would fly from Manchester to Dubai and then onto Perth. I went round to my Grandma's to tell her of my decision to leave University. I was a little worried as I thought she would be disappointed. She wasn't and was very supportive, she told me that

"Travel broadens the mind and you should not do something if it is making you unhappy".

I was pleased to have her blessing for my exploration. I decided to start off in Perth as a good friend of mine, Matthew, was out there playing cricket for six months. Matthew was a good drinking friend from school and sixth form. So the flight was booked, I told University that I would be leaving. I financed my trip mainly on savings and partly using the student loan I never spent. Richard and Tom took me to the airport, I was buzzing all the way thinking about what I was embarking on and my pals were also equally excited for me, or maybe they were just pleased I was leaving them for a while. I was so disorganised, I literally packed my bag on the day we were going to the airport, loaded my iPod with music and set off to Manchester. I pretty much lived my life that way, last minute, no plans, it will be alright in the end.

It just so happened that I booked the flight for a time when my Mum and Dad were on holiday, they don't believe me when I say this, they think I did it so it was them saying bye to me and not me saying bye to them. Once again it was just like when I started University on both occasions, I was full of ambition. I thought I was going to get there, meet the girl of my dreams, emigrate, get a fantastic job, go surfing every day and have BBQs all the time. So once again I set myself up for a massive fall as all of the above were unattainable. I sold my scooter the day before I left and I garaged the Polo GT and my pit bike in Peter's garage. I had a leaving party at the Yellow Lion and only Tom attended however I didn't promote it greatly.

I flew with Emirates and it was a lovely plane, it was practically empty and I had 3 seats to myself so I put my feet up and created a bed like position. I thought this is it, maybe I've cracked it. My worries seemed so far away and for the first time in ages I just felt at ease with life. This however all evaporated as soon as I stepped off the plane and the whole experience of leaving University and leaving home hit me and I started to panic a little. Like many things in life, the journey is often far greater than the destination. I got my bag and headed for the taxi rank. The driver asked me where I wanted to go and I said Perth, he said you're in Perth already! So I just ended up saying take me to where all the hostels were. He took me to Northbridge which was an area with a lot of hostels for travellers. The further we got from the airport the greater the nerves set in and the sinking feeling in my stomach descended upon me.

I got out of the taxi and put my rucksack over my shoulders and thought this is it time raise my weapons and fight. I went in a hostel for the first time in my life and asked if there were any rooms, he replied yes, it turned out it was to share with 12 people - I couldn't believe it, sharing with 11 other people. That wasn't for me I decided to go and find a hotel but got lost and ended up in the Central Business District, I went up to one hotel and asked them how much it was and it was something like $120 for one night. I thought I can't pay that and left. Now most normal people when they go travelling tend to book there first nights accommodation just so if they arrive at 3am in the morning on the other side of the world have somewhere to go. O no not I. I have to do it Tom's way, the 'it will be alright on the night' way. As I was walking around I kept seeing all the adverts for things to do and see and I started to think will I ever get to see these places, will I make any friends. I'm such an impatient person. I was back to how I felt in sixth form, Nottingham Trent and The University of Sheffield. This time I had no home to run back to no friends to comfort me, I had to make it work this time somehow. I ended up sleeping on a bench right next to the Swan River, I don't think I actually slept but I realised it wasn't going to be easy, I just was in a dazed sort of state I couldn't believe what had happened over the last few years and how now I was sat on a bench in Australia with a rucksack and absolutely fuck all else. What I did have was determination. I've never really been short of that. I then headed back to the backpacker area, I ended up going to a hostel called Mad Cats in Northbridge. It was rough, but seeing as it was my first experience I just thought this was normal. I only looked at the other hostels from the outside so it was hard to compare. It turned out that Mad Cats was the roughest hostel in Perth even possibly Australia. I shared a room with 11 other people and made friends with a nice chap called Ewan, he was Scottish and enjoyed a drink, maybe a little too much - even by my high levels of drinking and he realised eventually that he had a problem. We kept in touch and I went out to visit him a few times once we both got out of the hostels. I helped him with his CV and tried to help him find work, he was a steel fixer by trade and was a cracking guy. He was a nice man to chat too in my early days especially when I felt so alone. There was also a man than could hit a bottle so hard and with a special technique that the bottom flew of the bottle. I also got chatting to two Canadians, I can't remember both their names only one, Randy, I wonder why that one remained in my memory? She was lovely, I got chatting to them for a bit in my room, I really liked Randy. They told me they wanted to go to Broom, so as I was so keen to get with her I offered to take them to Broom. For starters I didn't have a car and secondly Broom was miles away. I probably should have got my atlas out before making such offers. It turns out driving from Perth to Broom is like driving from Dublin to Madrid. I just said I'd give them a lift there and drive home. Its not exactly like dropping your mate of in town. Anyway I told them I would take them but in the end I left them to it, they left before I got a car, probably a good job.

One thing Randy accidently left behind was a book called Scar Tissue by Anthony Kiedis. I grabbed it and stuffed it in my backpack. One day I took I out and started to read it. This was my first autobiography, now to say it was life changing is probably an overstatement but it certainly touched a nerve with me somewhere. The book basically talked about Keidis' battle with heroin and a whole host of other drugs and his raise to fame beating the odds. At the time of reading I was in a strange place in my life, I was new to Australia and didn't really know who I was or where I was heading. I was drifting along life's river with absolutely no control or direction. I was very easily influenced by other people and just wanted to be somebody and I didn't care how I got there. The book was an amazing story, I started to listen to his music and I absolutely loved it, I kind of felt something in common with him, I'm not sure what now but that's the feeling I had at the time. So here I was - my current role model was a rock star who had been addicted to Heroin. Just like back in the UK I had Mike Skinner.

After about 3 weeks of constantly going out with a few people from the Hostel I wasn't really making much progress mentally and was just feeling very alone and drinking to compensate for that feeling. There were a lot of tough characters in this hostel, mainly Ozzies who were working in Perth. Not the sort of people travellers like me was going to make friends with. One night I remember a few from the hostel went out drinking in Northbridge and I tagged along. It was an ok night but as usual I felt totally isolated. The next thing I knew was they had all left me, I was gutted. I just felt so unwanted and at a serious low point. My inner strength was immense back then, I just kept going. Although I felt deep sadness deep down I just buried it deep within me. I'd then brush myself down and formulate a new plan. Matt was about 30 minutes away from Perth where I was but I told myself before I went out there that I wouldn't bother him and that due to my insecurities felt he wouldn't have wanted to see me. In the end I put all those doubts to the back of my mind as I knew I needed to see a familiar face. I got in touch with Matthew via email, he didn't respond for a few days and I thought he didn't want to see me and I started to feel even worse. In the end we spoke via email and I arranged to meet him. We first hooked up on a day when he was playing cricket, he picked me up from the train station in Fremantle and we went to his cricket ground in Melville. It felt like such a weight had been lifted from my shoulders when I saw them and I relaxed a little. As Matt was playing cricket I sat with his girlfriend Sarah and drank far too many VBs (Victoria Bitter), we had a great day chatting and watching the cricket, Sarah is a lovely girl and we got on great, once the drink was in me I was talking some absolute rubbish. I felt on top of the world, such a contrast to how I was feeling days previous, this was probably due to the fact I was drinking a lot but mainly due to the company I was now under. But I felt at ease with life, I was free, I had a few quid in the bank and all my problems seemed miles away this despite the pretty rubbish start to my trip and the fact that I hadn't made any real friends as yet. I felt happiness or what I perceived happiness to be at that time in my life. Looking back its because I had ran away from my issues, the problem I had with regards been accepted by my piers or being popular been removed as I had no piers. At the time that was one of my biggest hang ups, plus I just didn't like myself at that time. But the answer to life's problems isn't to keep running, no one can run for ever and eventually they catch up with you.

Sarah probably had a few days left with Matthew and then it was just me and Matthew. Once Sarah had gone we hit the booze hard, two crates would last us one night and there would be a few left over, we were just constantly pissed! I remember going round to Matt's house in Melville and sitting on his veranda one evening in our early days together. We just sat there for hours talking complete bollocks and generally having the time of our lives. Matt's incredibly good company and we laughed a lot around that time. In the end I kind of moved into Matt's house for a while and lived on the floor in a spare bedroom. We'd just get up and go to the beach or go have a look at something somewhere. Perth is a lovely city and very different to the East Coast, there's a lot less there. There are some lovely places to eat however we never ate out, I lived of Subways and most days had 2 feet of them. However once I was with Matthew we cooked some good meals and ate much healthier. When I arrived in January the weather was incredible, the sun shone every day for months, it was very warm, touching the 40s.

It was around this time that I found out my old friend Skinner would be playing the Big Day Out in Perth so I went along on my own. I think the ticket was $140 but just before the event I managed to loose my ticket but I was so keen to see him that I paid again. I thought he's come all the way to see me. It was a good day as far as going to a festival on your own goes. I once again did my usual Mike/Tom relation trick but the Aussie chicks were not buying it.

To have the opportunity to be in Australia and see how they live when I was only 19 is something I am very grateful for. It would never have come about though should I have not had such bedlam going on within my head.

8. RANDOM STORIES OF LITTLE SIGNIFICANCE

I remember one session we had was at an away cricket match where Matt was playing, I left my car in the car park and went out. We ended up going to Fremantle but I lost Matt. I must have got a taxi to the cricket pitch as I remember waking up Saturday morning in the car park with all these kids pointing at me and hovering round my car. I was under a towel and it took me a few minutes to come round. It was certainly a strange way to be woken up. There were many of these sorts of nights and I had an absolute ball. Matt was great company, we had no worries all we wanted to do was have a good time. The Ozzies love their Sunday sessions and we did a few of them, a great place in Perth to go on a Sunday was Cotteslow Beach, lots of people would gather in the bars down there and it was a fantastic place to be in the world. The sun never stopped shining and the beers never stopped flowing. Maybe this was it? Maybe I had finally found happiness? The times me and Matthew shared in those early days of my time in Australia where some of my happiest memories, the fun we had was insurmountable and the memories I have will stay with me forever.

One of Matt's cricketing friends was having a house party and I was invited. We went round to this mans house and he was a very wealthy man and the house was amazing. We had a few bottles and the night got underway, it was a lovely warm summers evening and everyone was outside. After I'd had around 6 bottles I wandered over to this garage where a few of them were congregated. They were all stood around a bucket smoking. I went up to the group and said *"what's going on here then lads"* in my usual cocky way. They explained they were using a water bucket to smoke cannabis. I can't really remember the engineering behind it but basically it was a bucket full of water, a plastic bottle and some hose pipe used to inhale the fumes. They did something and it created a difference in pressure and somehow produced the fumes to which you smoke. They offered me a go to which I said yes and they said have you done this before as its strong and I responded with *"Yeah I do this sort of thing all the time"*. So I put my mouth around this pipe and waited and then all of a sudden this group of crazy Aussie's all started to shout "suck it in, breath in" and get very excited. I sucked as much as I could do then exhaled. Well nothing much happened and I asked for another go, I said it hadn't worked and that I needed another blast. They were a little concerned but one of the lads *said "he's cool man, he's done this loads of times back home"* so I went for my second session. Well fuck me. After a few minutes it hit me and I was in a serious mess. My mouth was watering and I felt extremely strange. I went up to Matthew and tried to talk but words were struggling to come to me. I looked at Matt and said *"I'm having an out of body experience"* I'll never forget saying those words to Matt in the garden. As I looked forwards the whole inside of my body was being twisted 90 degrees to my left. It was if somebody was turning a cog. It was such a strange experience. By this point I felt very poorly. I had to sit down, so I went into the cinema and there were big seats so I sat down in front of a massive screen and there was some Australian Football on. I sat there and my body went incredibly heavy, then what proceeded can only be described as a rollercoaster ride like no other. My body was pulling G's. All of a sudden I would be glued to the chair and I couldn't pull my body from it, it was being forced down by something. I got the feeling in my stomach when you go down a steep section on a ride, then it would be released. But I couldn't get out of the chair. I felt sensations in my body that I haven't felt before and probably will never feel again. It was a very fighting experience. There was a point when I nearly told Matthew to call an ambulance because I honestly believed I was going to die.

Matthew headed back to the UK after we had about 3 months together. While he was in Australia we managed to get some work in a meat works called Western Meat packers, it was here I appreciated the trade of a butcher, these lads in the works cut a side of beef up in seconds and it was amazing to see especially with my Dad being a butcher. My job was holding the rib so that they could cut down through the ribs with a circular saw. Matt's job was to sweep up!! Again we made the most out of it. The heat when you came out of the factory nearly knocked you off your feet as the factory was chilled. There was a grim smell about the place, I'm not sure what death smells like but I dare say it wasn't far from that. We only worked there for a week or two and then we went on a little road trip to a place called Monkey Mia, Shark Bay and the Pinnacles, this is a place about 1200 kilometres North of Perth. I drove for 12 hours straight with the assistance of Red Bull, Matt was supposed to drive as well but he fell asleep. There is literally nothing outside of the CBD, no villages or any sign of life. I drove for those 1200 KMs and literally saw a vehicle every hour. In Oz there are road trains and these are basically 3 trailers on a lorry. Rather an impressive site to see. The Pinnacles are spectacular rock formations that have eroded over time to create a great visual. We had a fantastic few days, we both slept in my car for most of the time and had BBQ's in the middle of nowhere. It felt like a proper adventure. We stayed in a hostel for the odd night. We missed the chance of seeing the dolphins at Monkey Mia as we were both too hung over but apart from that the little trip was a great success. One night we were staying in a bedsit type place and whilst under the influence we decided to put the whole of the contents of this bedsit into my car, when we woke up we couldn't believe what had happened, we thought we had been robbed until we walked out and saw the car with the fridge and bedside table amongst other things in it. It was the same night that someone had put vegemite under my door handles on the Falcon, so when I went to open the door my fingers got covered in the stuff. Guess that's good old Karma weaving her magic. While we're on the topic of my Falcon this car was a Ford and had a 4 litre straight six engine, it was automatic and was a dream to drive. I used to cruise everywhere in it with my Just Jack CD blasting out!

Before departing on our little adventure up North we and Matt had a little accident. We were both drinking the TEDs (Tooheys Extra Dry) and as ever they were going back nicely. We were both staggering about the garden in Melville and I became a little peckish. Previous to this point we had been eating Dominos pizzas almost every night. So I suggested about getting a Dominos. So we had a little debate about who should drive and Matt agreed to drive, I wanted to get a taxi. So we both fell into his Toyota Corona which without being disrespectful to Matt was somewhat of a relic. It was a 1987 2.0 auto! So he selects reverse and we navigate of his drive without a problem. We then start chatting away as we did, some random shite. We made it to Dominos, gets our pizza's and heads back down the highway back into Melville. So were trucking along, not talking at this point, the next thing is BANG, we smashed into the barrier in the middle of the road the bounced off the railings towards the gutter. Then we came to a stand still. Now I then proceeded to fall about in absolute hysterics it was the funniest thing. Matt on the other hand was shouting something like 'I can't believe it' and banged the steering wheel. Luckily though the pizzas where still intact. We got out of the car to assess the damage and once again a laughing outbreak erupted. It was a complete mess. We hit the front end on the barrier and made a serious mess of it, the car then spun and hit the opposite rear quarter on the other barrier. At this stage in Matt's life it was an extremely important asset to him. So we drove it home or should I say limped it home. The wheels were rubbing on the wings and it made an horrendous noise. The next week was operation salvage the Corona. Now this car was without a shadow of a doubt a right off however Matt couldn't deal with this fact so we repaired it. So you have to imagine this car wouldn't look out of place in a scrap yard, well in fact that's where it belonged. So Matt then buys a new indicator lense and proceeds to fit it. So we had a lump of metal with a nice shiny new indicator. Which flashed really quickly as all the others was smashed. We then thought it would be a good idea to straighten up the front end of the car. So we went and bought some heavy duty rope. There was a good strong tree in Matt's garden so we tied the rope around the front bumper and round the tree. Matt then got in the car and slammed it in reverse and attempted to straighten up the front end. Another truly comical moment, your friend realigning the front end of his car with a tree. In the end Matt gave me his car and I scrapped it. I've still got the keys somewhere.

It was time for Matt to leave and I took him to the airport, a funny little story was he had all these bags packed and they were crammed full. Anyway I went into the departures with him and he went to the check in desk and they said he was x amount over the limit and that he would have to pay so much to send it home. Well Matt decides to put all his cricket pads on and go through customs looking like Kevin Pietersen!! I took some off his other possessions home with me including about 8 cricket balls. I was sad to see him go, he was my only friend in Australia. I was now in a continent and I knew not one person. That's a very strange feeling but also very exciting.

I now needed somewhere to stay as I didn't want to return to the hostels, well not for now. So I got myself a lovely little ground floor flat which I shared with a women called Nina, this was located in a nice seaside resort called Scarborough. It was about a 15 minute drive from Perth but had a very nice feeling about it and the beach was amazing. My first job after Matt left was working in a dog food factory on the outskirts of Perth, my role here was basically taking the bags of food from the conveyer belt and placing them on a pallet, I would then wrap the whole lot in plastic filming. It wasn't a bad job actually and the people were great, the boss offered me a full time job but I turned it down. One time the machine broke down and this resulted in dog biscuits being projected into the air creating a dog biscuit type of rain. Very strange situation to be in but I'm sure is a Labradors dream.

While I was working there something rather strange happened. I worked very closely with a man on the conveyor belt, his job was to hold the bag under the funnel and fill it up with food and then seal it with a heating element. This lad was a bit of a character. He did however share many characteristics of my Uncle Mark and as time went on the more I thought about it there more I saw other mannerisms very similar to my Uncles. Until one day he was talking I actually thought it was my uncle. Now I obviously knew it wasn't but it was just so surreal. It was like my uncle had transported himself into another being near me just so he could see how I was getting on and let me know he was there. Very odd. My Uncle Mark gave me great inspiration to go to Australia as he too has travelled there amongst other places. It made me think, are the strangers we meet and talk too everyday strangers at all or is there something more too it than that. Are there only a certain number of people in the world and the rest you see are just images? Could the beautiful women we see from time to time actually be angels? I don't believe everything we see is actually real.

My next job was working in a town called Muchea which was about an hour North of Perth, the job was with a firm called Hay Australia. By this time I already had my fork lift truck licence and my role here was loading a bale of hay onto a conveyor belt, the hay went through the machine and came out the other end in small cubes and they were then sent to Japan. I met a great chap from Newcastle and he showed me the ropes. At the end of the shift I would have to climb in the machine where the razor blades were that cut the bales and pull out any twining that had got caught up. The job was actually too far away and my gas guzzling Ford Falcon used far too much fuel but I enjoyed the work. One problem with the job was that I have hay fever and I never thought about that when I applied – it was a disaster! I used to get in a right mess and had to physically pull my eyes open in a morning when I woke up in order to see anything. When I was at work I had goggles, masks and all sorts including shed loads of anti histamine to try and stop the irritation. In the end I decided I wanted something closer to Perth and in a job which had no relation to Hay! I got a bit of temporary work in a very prestigious casino in Perth called the Burswood as a fork lift driver. I didn't know at the time but they required an experienced forky but they sent me who had about 2 months experience and that was shifting hay bales. So I rocked up and there was this massive room and they were putting up these massive bi folding doors. There were about 10 lads 1 fork lift truck and me. So I gets there and they give me a brief on what they wanted doing and they were asking me all these technical questions which I didn't have a clue what the answers were. I was shitting it, I had to lift the doors up horizontally to a certain height then the lads would release the doors and they would spin 90 degrees to a vertical position. From there I would guide the doors in and some more lads on scissor lifts would fasten the doors in place. But the room for error was near enough none existent. There were chandeliers to avoid and very little space as doors by nature fit in a very small area. All the lads proper digged me for my skills, the site manger would often tell me how good I was. I was really pleased with myself and felt very fulfilled. Unfortunately this work was only temporary and once I had fitted the doors I was surplus to requirements but I had very happy times down at the casino.

It was around these early day in Scarborough that I first discovered Facebook, Matt told me about it when I was with him and I thought it was a bit geeky. So I left him too it and didn't think anymore about it. Then one night I was down the internet café and I signed up to it. It didn't take long before I was hooked. I used to go down the café every night from that point. I just kept adding friends and then adding more friends, I even got a message pop up that I was adding too many friends. Then I uploaded all my pictures and painted this wonderful image of myself. I was one of the first people to go travelling around my area and I wanted to show how good it was. That the thing with Facebook it makes you think everyone is having such an amazing life when in truth they probably aren't. It's often the opposite. So my life story to the world started right there in Scarborough.

9. ICE ICE BABY

I ended up getting a job working for a small building company where I worked at several sites and the company was owned by a man and a woman, they were a lovely couple but their son, who also worked there was a bit of a dick. I worked with them for 6 weeks or so then managed to land a job as a brick layers labourer for an English guy from Brighton called Steve. He was fantastic, I should never have got the job as I had no experience but he was desperate as he had been let down by more experienced labourers and gave me a chance. Previous to this I rang another advert up for an experienced labourer, I told the guy I had experience and thought what can there possibly be to know about being a brick layers labourer. I was wrong, I arrived there at 7am and he said 'make us a mix' to which I asked 'can you please tell me how to do that' then of course it was clear I did not have any clue what to do. He told me to leave but kindly gave me $20. So I started with Steve, I must admit I wasn't the best labourer but I got by. He worked in a gang of four and all the lads were great even though I got some stick for being a Pommy and also because I often cocked up. I remember one time Steve said to me;

"You know you Tom, everything you touch turns to shit".

That's because I somehow managed to break the cement mixer for a second time. We all used to have a few beers after work sat around in the building site, often the work was located by the sea so we had great views. The winter in Perth was a pretty bad one by their standards and as we were working outside we often were rained off. As I had no friends at this point I didn't really know what to do with myself, much of my time was spent in Perth wandering around the streets or in the shopping malls. I guess I just tried to do things rather than just sit about. The lads always used to go into the TAB (which is an Australian bookies that sell alcohol) and watch racing and drink so I would sometimes accompany them. There were a lot of nice days though especially towards the end of summer and I would often wonder down the beach in Scarborough on my own. It was a lovely spot and there would sometimes be weddings going on down there. I found a lot of contentment down the beach next to the sea, I found it very peaceful just watching the waves roll over. As this was on the West coast the sun would set in the sea and I would without fail go and watch the sunset every night I could. I suppose it was my soap opera and it certainly beat watching telly.   I was strangely rather happy around this time although I had very little contact with other humans. After reading Scar Tissue I read so many autobiographies, there was even a book shop in Scarborough and one of the books I bought was about Ronnie Biggs. So I had the sunset, beer and a book and didn't really want anymore than that. I lost all my preconceptions about what I thought I needed to be happy and just got on with life.

Whilst I was working I went on a bit of a road trip with Martin, he was older than me and a bit of a character and had been in quite a lot of trouble back home in England and had to make an escape. I met Martin in a caravan park when I was living in my car just before Matt left. He was a very confident man and knew exactly what he wanted. I of course was not and kind of just went along with him. He was a good bloke and he had some amazing stories, he knew a lot about life and had seen a lot and had been in some tricky situations. So we first met in the caravan site near Fremantle, we used to BBQ every night and just chill out listening to Morcheeba. Shortly after Matt left we headed south from Perth visiting all the sites along the way. The places were beautiful along the way and a lot Greener. The seas were also very blue and we went to a site where the two great oceans meet. There was a place called Margaret River and we did a tour one day around a vineyard which was amazing. The scenery was just phenomenal and I really felt like I was seeing the world. There were little shops on these vineyards that sold all different types of cheese and you could just sample as much as you like. It was a really high class area. This one night we ended up in a small town called Bundbury where we stayed on a caravan park which had a lake on site which was very nice. We got settled in and cooked some tea on the gas BBQ's that were there. We had our meal and had a few beers and decided to head out into town. We went to a bar and it was full of Ozzies, not surprising I know given the fact we were in Australia. So we carried on drinking and chatting and this girl walked into the bar. Martin approached her and was giving her all the chat. She drifted away and Martin came back to me and we talked again to each other. Martin, who knew a lot about the drug scene said that the girl was definitely on something. I thought no more about it and carried on drinking. The girl retuned to the bar and Martin talked some more to her. He then told me that he was right and she was actually of her rocker on crystal meth.

She was leaving and all three of us left the bar together, by this point it was the end of the night and I'd had a lot to drink and was fairly drunk. We called at the bottle shop and bought a crate of Tooheys New. She threw the crate over her shoulder and proceeded to march back to her place. She was wearing extremely short shorts and boots. We arrived at her place in this bizarre area somewhere on the outskirts of Bunbury. The house was very small and dirty and she shared it with her friend who had a baby. She pulled a bag out of her bra which contained the Meth. Her and Martin then sat down at a table and she picked up a light bulb. This bulb had the element removed from it and just left glass bulb. She then proceeded to sprinkle crystals into the bulb. The outer casing of a pen was used as a pipe, she then used the flame of lighter to heat the crystals, her other hand covered the top of the bulb so no gasses could escape. Once enough smoke was created and the crystals were gone she created a small hole for the pipe to slot into. It was then inhaled like a cigarette. The exercise was then repeated for Martin. I was massively fascinated by this however declined the offer to try it. I just had a beer and watched. They had another round with the Ice and I was offered a go once again. I declined but then for some reason I took them up on the offer. I sat there while the girl heated the bulb up with the pen in my hand, my heart was pumping like crazy and I was scared. She told me to put in the pen and suck as hard as I could. I did this, I just kept on breathing until my lungs couldn't take anymore of this substance. I held it in for a few seconds and let it circulate with body, I then slowly expanded my lungs and allowed this drug to smoothly come out of my lips and into the room. Nothing happened at first, there was a pause, then it hit me: BANG. The best way to describe the feeling is by putting A Sky Full of Stars on from Coldplay's Ghost Stories album – the slight pause is important. An intense feeling of clarity took over my brain and I had arrived. My mind and body became one and I was immensely sharp. I knew exactly what I wanted and how I was going to get it. I had no doubt in my brain, there was no second guessing, and everything was simple. I wouldn't stop talking, my brain was just on overdrive I had all these ideas and I just wanted to tell everyone. I needed more. I'd had quite a big hit but I needed another one. Just like with drinking I was greedy. The girl did me another one. We kept drinking and the feeling was powerful. Ecstasy is more of a happy loved up feeling but this was far greater far more direct and triggered a much greater chemical reaction within my brain. We had more, the poor girl ran out and she had to get her dealer round to give us some more gear, we didn't even have any money but we needed the substance now. I filled my lungs again with the swirling white clouds of magic and once again I went to another dimension.

We then left her house and tried to find our way back. Martin wasn't so bad but I was wired. My mouth was all dry and I kept moving my tongue around my teeth, I could taste the stuff in my mouth. I couldn't relax I was on edge, I needed to keep walking my brain was working overtime and I didn't know how to stop it. Martin went back to the site but I couldn't sleep. I got my phone out and proceeded to ring everyone in my phone. Literally everyone. I couldn't stop talking, I didn't give them chance to respond. I rang Christine who I used to work with and she said to me whilst on the phone to stay of the drugs, I think she knew what I had been up too.

I walked around this lake probably 3 times and topped my phone up 2 times. It was light when I returned to the caravan site, I went over and banged on Martins van to talk some more rubbish. We owed the girl something like $120 and we had agreed to pay her. Martin asked if I wanted to not pay her but I insisted we did. It was the least we could do plus she owed it her dealer and could have got in a lot of trouble. We set of driving and randomly met up with this shy lad from England, I was still out of my tree and yet again talked some more rubbish and Martin in the end had to tell me to shut up. The feeling of confidence and clarity left me probably around midday. Then came the feelings of guilt about taking the drug and the fear of the consequences. I then ran through all the conversations I had had and again that filled me with dread. It felt like my stomach had been tied in a knot. I didn't know what to do, we were in a little fishing village further south called Busselton which had a long pier. Anyway the come down hit me. The high was immense but like everything it came with a cost, the feeling of utter self-worthlessness was incredible, all of the negativity within my body festered up and hit me like a truck. However I told myself it was my gap year to do whatever I felt was right. You will have your own views as to whether this was morally right or wrong but I had chosen my path and wasn't in a position to turn around. Plus don't you have to do all these crazy things to be somebody?

The whole experience was amazing and Martin and I knew we would have to try that again. We continued further down South and reached Albany, there wasn't much further past Albany and the next destination along the coast was too far so we returned to Perth. I returned to work and me and Martin kept in contact, we managed to find a supplier of crystal meth in Perth and we would go to a car park just out of town and buy some. On one occasion we headed back to Scarborough with the gear and went round the back of the Commonwealth Bank where I used to do my banking. Martin had prepared some strips of tin foil and once again we were creating those swirling pools of smoke that found their way into out bodies. The feeling again was amazing and we headed off to a bar in Scarborough to watch a jazz band, the night was fantastic.

After I had worked for a while I managed to save a decent amount of money up. I treated myself to a motorbike, I bought a Honda CBR 600F, and it was a 1998 model. From memory it cost around $5,000. I used to go for rides after work on my own and try and find some windy roads, the problem with Perth was, as it was relatively new the roads were straight but out in the hills you could get your knee down a little. I at the time was very silly in regards to my safety. Once my confidence grew I tried to ride harder and faster and push myself. I'm not saying I was a fantastic rider but I began to know the bike and my own limitations and as normal pushed it.

I would often head down to Rockingham where Martin was living with his uncle. We used to go to his local pub called the Wacky which was very rough and full of real Aussies so much so that when they talked to me in the toilets I'd talk back with an Australian accent. There must be something in the water in Australia as those lads certainly knew how to grow a beard. We sourced some amphetamine's to add some spice to our nights. This was less powerful than the ice however my senses became immensely heightened and my confidence increased. Just like other drugs a mist of clarity came over my brain and I became in the moment once again. There were no worries holding me back and all doubt had gone. It was great riding my motorbike home back to Perth the next morning, the drug was still in my system and my confidence and skill at riding was greatly intensified. Mixing speed on the road and speed in the brain results in a different kind of feeling. While in the hostels a few lads used to go on about how good the ecstasy was over in Australia and that it was much better than back home in England. They cost around $20 at the time which was incredibly expensive compared to England where they were typically about £1 each. It was said that you would only need one, I guess like it used to be in England when ecstasy first become popular. So we purchased our pill and we decided to have half each and mix it with some speed and a few drinks. We were massively disappointed as the little cocktail did nothing too us. We just felt very disappointed especially when we were expecting this amazing feeling to come over us. It may have been a bad batch. Drugs are very unreliable and you cannot guarantee the same feeling again and again. The good feeling was non existent compared with the time in Gatecrasher but that's probably due to the fact I'd 17 back home. Luckily I didn't chase the buzz and left it. Eventually the highs aren't as good as they were the first time and that's where the problems start, eventually your body becomes used to the drug and produces chemicals to counter balance the drugs desired effect. It was on one of these chemical fuelled nights that I fell in love with a stripper called Ashley. She was an Australian girl and was very attractive. I talked to her a bit and she complemented me on my accent which really isn't really a compliment at all. Anyway she gave me her number and I liked her that much I wrote it down in my passport. Its still in now but heavily crossed out. I waited all of the next day to ring her and I had it all mapped out what I was going to say. I was at the races in Perth and was very excited to make the call. I went to one side and rang her. It didn't even ring. The number was the wrong one. I couldn't believe it, I was gutted.

10. SPEED OVERDOSE

One time I went to meet Martin. We had a cracking night and we had a beer in a beer garden one lovely evening in Fremantle, I ended up having probably 3 pints and then I left Martin to head back to my place in Scarborough. For some reason I decided to give the bike a bit of poke and see how fast it went, I wound the revs on and my head was down under the windscreen. I just kept my wrist in the same position. I decided to have a quick look at the speedo as I wanted to know how fast I was doing. The last figure I remember seeing was 240 km/h but I just kept on going. I was like a rocket being projected down the Scarborough Beach Highway, I was now a pillion and had no control whatsoever. I kept up the speed all the way until I had to come of the highway and turn up my street towards my flat. I was still giving it all I had and pulled up at my flat. My adrenaline when I got off the bike was immense and I felt buzzing. The next thing I knew a police car pulled up behind where I had parked my bike. The lights were blazing and I remember thinking this was like something from Neighbours. All the curtain twitches were out in full force that evening. There were 2 policemen, they said do you know how fast you were doing? I of course denied that I did. They informed me that I shot past them on the highway and they were unable to record my speed. It was an unmarked police car. They then put me in the back of the police car and asked me further questions. As a matter of course they breathalysed me, I knew I had had a couple of pints but thought I was going to be ok. I wasn't actually sure what the legal drink drive limit was in Australia. I waited in anticipation whilst the results were being calculated on the machine. A Red light came up, my stomach sank and I innocently asked what the Red light was for, naturally they informed me it was a fail and I was duly arrested. I was then taken to Northbridge police station in Perth. All I was bothered about in the car on the way down to the station was whether or not by having such a conviction would affect my chances of becoming a resident. The policemen were alright with me and we chatted a little. My adrenaline was even higher at this point and I guess so were the nerves. They took me into the station and eventually I was taken to a room where they completed a full test and I think they even did a test on me for opiates. I kept the print out to show my Mum in case she ever wondered if I'd been dabbling in a spot of heroin. I produced my licence and after some more time in the station I was released and I think I was told I'd receive the charges in the post. I got out of the station and was still buzzing, I felt like I did back in Loughborough, I felt like I was living. Now I'm older I know that is a strange reaction to have for a serious crime but all I wanted to do was be more interesting. Obviously it doesn't and I know many people who have been arrested for drink driving and I think there are silly. But I was 19 and in Australia so what happened over there didn't count. Or so I believed.

A few weeks passed and I received a chunky letter through the letter box, I opened it and it was from the courts I think. I read the paperwork and was horrified. I had been charged with drink driving, driving without a licence and reckless driving. This was serious. It was all official and suddenly my actions now carried consequences. The description of what I had done was very exaggerated and did make my actions appear far worse than the facts. However the truth was I had done wrong and committed a crime. The court date was set.

Shortly after purchasing my bike I sold the falcon and bought a Nissan Micra which was by all intents and purposes and shed. It was even below the class of Matt's pre crash Corona. After my arrest I sold the bike, I didn't want anything to do with it. This just left me with the Nissan.

A few weeks passed after receiving my letter and the court date eventually arrived. I remember the morning of my court appearance, I was in the shower and I thought to myself I was either going to end up in court or end up in a box. I was just silly on the bike, something just used to take over my brain and I needed that fix of speed. Every rational thought in my head of my wellbeing disappeared in an instance and I would enter into this third dimension. There is no excuse for it but once you have had your fix like any addiction you want it again. For me speed was like meditation, there was nothing in my brain just the tarmac that lay ahead of me. No worries about who I was or where I was heading existed anymore, instead there was just a crystal clarity that is very hard to find.

I used to ride it everywhere in shorts and a t shirt although on the night of my arrest I had jeans on. I decided against having a lawyer due to the cost. There was a duty lawyer available on the day for a small cost of $20 who I did see before my hearing. In my defence the lawyer thought reckless driving was a little harsh given the facts. She advised me that I should appeal the charge. She also informed me it carried a maximum sentence of 2 years imprisonment and that really shocked me. It was starting to become real, what happens if the judge believes I deserve a prison sentence? My attitude to the whole episode was very blasé and I remember not worrying, I just remember thinking this will make a good story for the lads back home. I don't worry about the big things in life but I worry immensely about the small things such has how I come across or what people think, I guess I'm backwards. It's impossible for me to believe this now but I can assure I had very little fear around this time in my life. Although the prison sentence was in the back of my mind I wasn't even too bothered about that, I thought it would make me more interesting and add something unique to my life.

I went into the court room and there were a lot of people in attendance. The 2 police officers from the night of my offence were present as well as other people who I didn't really know where there. Again I was buzzing, the spot light was on me and I liked that. We were all sat down and the judge walked in and we were all told to rise, I didn't realise this as I was in my own little world. So a lady to the left motioned at me to stand up by raising her palm in an upwards fashion. So we were all stood up.

The judge was a lady and had ginger hair, she read out all the charges one by one which sounded very bad. Then the policemen gave their evidence and went through in great detail what I was accused of doing. Once everyone had talked the judge asked me

"How do you plead"

I replied

"Guilty but I'm not guilty"

She said you can't say that so I said

"I plead guilty as I'm heading off up North and can't prolong my sentencing".

The judge was baffled by such a comment, I was showing of. I was arrogant and wanted to portray to the courtroom that I wasn't intimidated by them. Cocky kid from Sheffield sticking his middle finger up to the Australian criminal justice system or so he thought.

After a while of deliberating my sentence was handed down to me. I was fined $1,400 and banned from driving for 1 year - luckily no prison sentence. In Australia there is a sliding scale for drink driving and not a straight ban, as I was only just over the limit I just received a fine, my ban was for reckless driving. With regards to the driving without a licence element of the conviction I did have a full motorbike licence but never updated my photo card before leaving the UK, it still showed that I was restricted to 33bhp and of course my bike was well over that. I could have contacted the DVLA and got them to fax over the updated licence and this would have helped my plea however I left it too late and never did anything.

I sold the Micra and now had no vehicles, my empire of automobiles had fallen and I was left with the very dirty, unreliable and over priced public transport system. Steve who I was working for kindly offered me a place in his house with his family as he knew I wouldn't be able to get to work. I took him up on it. Things weren't working out with Benny and Carol who I was living with back in Scarborough and it was time to move on, plus I could get to work. Steve and I had a fantastic 4 weeks together and I really got to know him as a person. He was very comical and would often have me in fits of laughter. He was originally from Brighton but emigrated to Australia with his wife when he was very young. He worked as a bricklayer back home in England and eventually set up a business in Perth. He had a lovely house with a swimming pool and a games room in a nice suburb of Perth. Steve and his wife lived there with their 3 children who were all very welcoming. The gang of lads at work were great as I said, they would have what's called a smoko. This was an hour and in this time they would all play games for money, it was extremely good fun. Some games we used to play were so interesting and creative. One time Steve thought of a new game called 'chase the ace' which included a large board with a load of pins attached too it and some cards. The game was going to last a long time and required each day one person to pick a card and if it matched the card (An ace I guess?) selected then they would receive the money. Anyway Steve spent ages pinning all the cards up and buying the board etc. I was by this point already living at Steve's house. We took this massive board which was his pride and joy into the site and stuck it in the corner. Everyone was excited to start the game as there would eventually be some big money riding on it. It was agreed that I would be the first person to pick the card. I made my selection and pulled the card from the board. It was the winning card. The lads couldn't believe it, they were adamant that I had cheated. They knew I was staying at Steve's and had access to the garage. I couldn't believe it, what a twat I felt, I didn't know what to say. What were the chances of that? I tried to give back the winnings but they wouldn't have it. Instead a blew the $100 on the TAB. Everyone was well and truly pissed off with me.

Before I moved in with Steve he would ask me every Monday morning "Have you had a root this weekend Tom" then of course everyone else would join in with the piss taking. They were happy days and I owe Steve a lot, he became a good friend in those months in Perth and I certainly like to think a small fraction of my personality derives from Steve.

Me and Steve would come home from work and get on the Toohey's Extra Dry. I think his wife got a bit fed up with us in the end as all we did was drink! I remember on more than one occasion been sat at the dinner table with the family and been in hysterics at Steve. I knew everyone was getting annoyed but it just made us laugh even more. It was Steve who introduced me to the book The Secret, I also saw it on a talk show over there and knew I had to buy it. The book basically describes the fact that you can obtain everything you want and desire in life by using your mind. I found it fascinating and thought the possibilities of life are endless. On one page there is an exercise and asks you to try really hard with your mind to imagine a free cup of coffee. You have to believe that you are going to receive a free coffee and feel what it is like to have it using all your senses. I was sat on Scarborough beach attempting this exercise then all of a sudden I hear this tune been played from what I thought was an ice cream van. I turned around to the car park that was behind me and it was a van giving away free samples of iced coffee. Now I was in shock. I had goose pimples all around me and just sat there. I didn't get up and have a coffee. This was just pure coincidence but what coincidence. The next thing I did was picture a beautiful woman coming to sit alongside me on the beach. Well the books good but not that good.

II. ALL THAT GLITTERS ISN'T GOLD

I met Benny when I was doing the building work on schools in Perth. I eventually moved out of my flat with Nina and moved in with him. He was a lot older than me and he was a very wise man. Before I moved in with him he and his now wife Carol were living next door after I had persuaded them to move to Scarborough. I told them Scarborough was this amazing place and they would love it too. I met Carol for the first time in a backpackers in Perth and we go on fantastic, there was plenty of wine flowing and I felt at ease with them both. I decided to move in with them as we had a good laugh and I wanted to be with people my own age and although Nina was nice she was probably in her 50's. While we are on the subject of Nina she invited me to her ex husbands Easter party. Now that was one of the most awkward days of my life. She told the guests who included her grown up daughters as well as her ex husband that I was living with her. She added very little information as to the circumstances of the actual relationship I had with Nina, which of course was land owner and tenant. The day seemed to last for ages and everyone thought I was a complete idiot. For obvious reasons her husband did not say one word to me and the whole event was silly and I should not have attended. However as always I thought it was a good idea at the time. She was a lovely women though and had a lot of time for me. When I first moved in she told me not to use the washing machine but instead to use the shared ones at the bottom of the drive. So of course I decided to use the one in the flat. Well I can only remember one item that I put in it and that was a dark Blue t-shirt and of course other items. So I put on the washing machine and thought no more about it. I walked back in the flat and there was a thin layer of Blue water throughout the flat. I just stood there in this rather large puddle. I had to use the mop and soak all the water up, it took ages. All the colours in my Blue t-shirt had all ran and it now resembled a greyish tone. Nina never find out about my washing day. I have since learnt to follow orders from middle aged women about kitchen appliances and listen to advice. People know more than me, a concept that I often find hard to grasp but I usually realise this at my cost.

So I moved out and in with the neighbours. The couple that replaced me in the flat were also Irish and crikey o riley the girl who's name I've forgot was absolutely out of this world. A strong 9 by anyone's standards and had a lovely personality to go with it. Her partner was a nice chap and probably made her very happy.

After living with Benny and Carol for a while Carol and I began to fall out and she took a slight disliking too me. Things were good at first but soon declined. She really regretted moving to Scarborough and as I had told them how good it was felt really bad. I can't really blame them for the decline in friendship as I used to be drunk a lot and I always talked during films which really annoyed them. I took this very personally as I really wanted to fit in with them and have a good time. Plus I also had a lot of admiration for Benny. I saw it as a big blow to my already small levels of self confidence. In the end we were discussing leaving Perth and up until this point I was going to travel around Australia with them but it was made clear to me that they would be travelling alone. Unfortunately we finished on bad terms which were a shame especially when things started off so well. Previous to the parting I was introduced to many of their Irish friends and we all used to go out however I felt so out of the circle, just like I was in University. Some of their friends were openly unpleasant and again crippled my already fragile personality.

It was whilst I was in Scarborough that I met a character called Pete, Pete was an older guy probably in his 70s at the time, he lived in the flat above me in Scarborough. He seemed like a really genuine guy and he took me to the races a few times and even lent Benny his Ute. He had a few stories, I'm unsure what was true and what wasn't but he said he used to have a boat and a pub but the pub was burnt down. Anyway I liked the guy and trusted him, he was always very helpful and I didn't have any reason not to like him. He called me up to his flat where he and he wife were sitting in the lounge. We got chatting and he offered me the chance to buy some shares in a gold mine. The shares were going on sale for 25 cents and he told me they'd be at $2.50 by Christmas which I thought would be great, I'd sell them and make a killing then I would then travel home via New Zealand and America and do some more travelling. I agreed that I would make the purchase of shares and met him in this car park where I was to go into the bank to withdraw the cash. I then got in his Ute (utility, like a pick up) and made the exchange. He then gave me a homemade receipt and we parted company. I didn't think anymore about my investment and looked forward to them being floated on the Australian Stock Exchange. Time passed and just before Christmas I rang Pete as I was struggling for cash and he told me they still hadn't gone on the market let alone make any profit. I bought $3000 worth of shares and it was my ticket home, but all I'd got was a scrappy piece of paper saying that I had purchased them. The shares in hindsight weren't even in my name and were for a company called Tasman Goldfields which I technically own part of. I've since been informed the company changed names. So with that and my fines I was nearly $5,000 down on my travelling fund. Thinking about it now I believe it was a con. I guess I'll never know but I'd love to go back to Scarborough and ask Pete whatever happened to my savings. Benny and Carol also bought some shares and in my paranoid head I often ponder as to who exactly were in on the con. I'll never know I guess but it was a very costly decision to make. I told a few mates back home and luckily for them and me they have half a brain cell and thought it sounded dodgy. I couldn't have dealt with loosing there money.

After a while of saving and working in Perth I decided I would leave Steve and his family and head North as I felt I was starting to out stay my welcome. I had seen the coast from Albany to Shark Bay and it made sense to fly, plus of course I didn't have a licence anymore. I left Perth around June time which was the middle of their winter, I had stayed much longer than I had planned in Perth but I had got settled and rather enjoyed my new life in Scarborough. Whilst I was in Perth there was a mining boom on and there was work for travellers everywhere, you could walk into an agency or look at a hostel notice board and people were chucking work at you. The money also was very good, I think a labourers wage when I was there which in 2007 was in the region of $18 per hour and using the exchange rate at the time of 0.40p to $1 meant I was earning just under £8. Now back home the minimum wage was probably £4.75 p/h for the same time period. The fuel in Australia was extremely cheap and you didn't have to insure your car as it was included in a payment known as rego. This covered you 3rd party. Food, drink and rent were very expensive meaning you weren't actually any better off, so it's all relative really. When I worked for Steve a good bricklayer's labourer was earning $200 a day and some firms paid more. This worked out as £400 a week and was a good wage. As my labouring skills were not so brilliant I think I was earning $140 a day. However as all of the work was outside we didn't ever get a week's work completed due to the weather. This affected my savings forecast considerably, in addition to this there was my gold mine investment, rather large fine, high levels of alcohol consumption and discovery of class A drugs. All this resulted in a significantly reduced spending budget. Luckily I had taken quite a bit of money out with me so I still had scope to make a move away from Western Australia.

I said all my goodbyes to Steve and his clan and got a cab to the airport, the last time I had been at the airport was to wave Matthew of through customs looking like his was walking out into a test match at Lords. This time it was my turn to jump on that big bird and commence my adventure into the unknown.

12. EMMANUELLE

The flight was in the evening and there was a fantastic sky, we hugged the side of the coast and left the lights of Perth city behind and headed to much dustier lands, the sun was setting in a scarlet sky. The flight lasted a couple of hours and we touched down in Broome at 19.25, it was dark and there were no skyscrapers or bright lights to look at. The terminal was hard to describe in Broom, it was a wooden building and was the size of a gymnasium hall. The customs officials were dressed in beige shorts, a white polo shirt and white socks that were pulled right up to their knees. They also had straw hats. I found this all very odd and it felt like I had stepped into a different country. Perth was a city and like all cities doesn't shock you much. All of our bags were chucked onto the big conveyor belt and I stood there looking at the conveyor going round and round. I was in a trance. One by one all of the people left the building and I suddenly realised I was the only one left. Where on earth was my bag? I just starred at the belt some more and there was just one bag left and I kept seeing it go past. But where was mine. In the end I went to tell one of these men who were stood to the side observing. He went over and pulled the last remaining bag of the carrousel and said is this yours sir. I said actually yes it is. He looked at me in a bizarre way, I said it was faced down and I've never seen my bag before faced down. So here I was, I had arrived. I checked into the hostel 'Broome's Last Resort'.

Everybody in Broome drove Landcruisers and had fuel canisters fastened to their roofs, this was due to the remoteness of the place and the fact that there were such great distances between gas stations. All the properties were single storey from what I remember and I believe some houses were on stilts. I met a lovely Scottish girl called Kirsty on my second day in Broome, we played table tennis and I let her win. We then went for a walk and sat and drank a few Corona's on a cricket pitch. My diary says 'I returned back to the hostel and by this point I was well pissed and collapsed. I woke up at 2am to find Kirsty had vanished'. You probably think I've got a massive diary for the time I was away however I don't unfortunately. I guess my lack of commitment and 'seeing things through to the end' beat me once again. The Diary of Tom Gray would maybe make an interesting read if not somewhat repetitive. I guess I didn't want to write the bad parts down, I wanted to portray a different experience.

Martin had been going to Thailand for 10 years when I met him and raved about it, everything was Thailand this and when I was in Thailand I did that. He really painted this amazing picture of the place and it sounded amazing. He was heading out there in August for a few months and asked me if I would go, I said it sounds great but I declined his offer. After some persuasion he eventually got me to book some flights. I decided I would fly out of Darwin and meet Martin in Phuket for 3 weeks. So the flights were booked and I now needed to get to Darwin from Broome in about 12 days however I had no plan in place and no idea of how I was going to do this. As it was winter in the South everyone had headed north to follow the sun just like myself, before I arrived in Broome I expected to walk into a hostel meet up with two lovely hunnies and catch a ride with them to Darwin. Just as easy as that. That unfortunately never happened, so I had to look elsewhere and construct plan B. I looked at flights but these were all booked, all the greyhound buses were booked and I didn't know what else to do. I wondered around Broome and I knew time was ticking, if I didn't make it to Darwin I would miss my flights. My diary says 'met a bloke called Pete who reckoned he was the boss of DHL, but now works in a bottle shop. Decent bloke but shit at pool.' I stayed a night at the Kimberley Klub ($27 a night) which was a much nicer hostel.

I found one last remaining option and it was by the way of an 'Ozzy Adventure' tour. You basically all jump on this giant bus and make your way to Darwin with a tour guide but you pay $1,535 for the pleasure. At this point in my life the idea of being stuck with 15 strangers on a bus for 10 days was my idea of hell. I couldn't do it. What would I say? How would I talk to these people in the day without having a drink? All of these negative thoughts were rushing around my head and I was in a panic. If I didn't go I'd miss my flights. If I went I would be forced to talk to strangers and make conversation without the luxury of being able to leave the situation as we would be stuck in one place. In the end I decided to go with the 'Fuck It' approach which had now become my default setting. Whatever was put in front of me I went for. Good or bad I did it.

We set of from Broome and I got myself right at the back of the bus and put on my music. I was so pissed off that it had come to this, I had the belief that only geeky travellers did these sort of trips and the cool kids like me cruised along the highway listening to Stereophonics Dakota with immensely attractive Scandinavian women. I however was on the bus and I was to stay on the bus. We drove for a while and then we stopped. I knew this was the moment, the time had come, I had to speak to a fellow citizen of the earth. This time there was no alcohol to aid me on my conquest into the unknown. I can't remember what I said but I began to ease up, only a little at first but I started to like it. This fed into me talking a little more and as the days passed I got to know each and everyone on the trip. The first site we saw was the Boab Prison Tree, this is a big tree where they used to put Aborigines. From there we went on to Winjana Gorge where we saw crocodiles. Then we had tea which was salmon cooked on the coals. We played the animal noises game which is exactly what it sounds like, you make animal noises but its amazing how different the noises are when different nationalities do it. Japanese were always the best.

There were people from all over Europe, Japan, Australia and other places. There were lawyers, doctors, students, travellers and many other varied and interesting occupations. I came out of my shell and I really enjoyed talking to these new people and learning about their lives and their cultures, they were fascinating and I got the feeling from a few of them that they actually liked my company. This was immensely valuable to me and was the main purpose behind my trip to Australia. I felt I was a different person to who I was in those hostels in Perth, I was me. Or a me I liked and wanted to keep.

Another place we visited was Tunnel Gorge where we went caving, then Bell Gorge, here there was a beautiful waterfall and plunge pool where we all went swimming. My diary says 'Had a few beers and tried to put the world to rights. This was interesting as there were English, Australian, German and Swedish'.

The next day we headed to Galvin Gorge. Everything was just Gorge-us. Get it? We then headed to the Bungle Bungles in the Purnululu National Park which are one of the most fascinating physical land formations I've ever seen, especially when the sun is going down.

We visited this most amazing place called El Questro, this is an exclusive hotel by Voyages and some rooms where $2,000 per night. There were some interesting people at the bar. The hotel is part of a million acre cattle station and everything is just stunning. We stayed one night and there were all these blokes singing, playing on guitars, dancing and drinking all around a big fire. Whilst at El Questro we visited Zebedee Falls which are a natural spring and the temperature of the water was 34 degrees. It was such a unique experience which I know not many people will ever experience. That to me was what travelling is all about, not cooped up in some concrete jungle chasing a false dream. We learnt a lot about the Aborigines people and had the chance to meet them. I saw all of their amazing art work that dates back a long time. These people live in some of the most horrendous conditions known to man while other people live in such amazing conditions in their wealthy cities. I was informed of a man who once wanted to poison these people, who I may add actually own the country, by putting something in their water. This wasn't centuries ago but just a few decades ago. The Aborigines have such amazing talents and have suffered greatly since their country was invaded. Of course not all of them are but what group of people are all good?

We also went onto Lake Argyle which is a very large lake, we took a boar trip and fed these fishes which squirt water at you. An incredibly poor story I must admit but I'll keep it in anyway for a bit of fun.

There were two French girls from Paris and I took a liking to one, Emmanuelle. We got on fantastic and I used to talk to the pair in French. Well what I actually did was say every single French word I had ever heard no matter what order or what context. My main memory from GCSE French was stationary equipment so I would often shout out very loudly 'glue stick' which girls just love to hear. They liked this and they laughed a lot and it added into my already good feeling of self worth. I tried my French speaking tricks with the English girls but it doesn't have the same impact. We become great friends and I liked her a lot, I wasn't sure what was going to happen but she told me she was leaving the tour early in a few days. One problem I have is I don't say how I feel, especially in this situation. I couldn't read it, I didn't want to attempt to make a move and for her to go crazy and be offended. I took my usual stance when it came to girls I liked and that was do nothing. She came onto the bus and said bye and that was it. She was gone forever. Well she thought she had seen the last of me until I hunted her down on Facebook. I added her as a friend and she gave me some story that she didn't want her ex boyfriend to find out about me. Another lessoned learned, if you like someone tell them as they may disappear from your life for good. I still wouldn't know what to do if I was in the same situation.

Again it was drinking every night and eating round a camp fire, we would have a massive pot and cook stuff in the fire from kangaroo to fish. We weren't staying on proper sites so we had to use the things we had. We saw some great landscapes and the scenery was fantastic and after been stuck in a city for so long it was a total culture shock. Before I left Perth I bought myself some Nike TN's in White, I told the lady I was heading to Broome and she said they wont stay White long due to the red sand, I thought she was pulling my leg. They stayed White for about 10 minutes.

I was so pleased to be making new friends and having fun, all my worries of fitting in seemed to disappear and I was in my element. It was an experience I'll never forget and I met some inspiring people. It was such a great feeling of becoming closer to the person I wanted to be after what seemed like a long time not been.

So we rocked up at Darwin, the group went out for tea and we had a great time all chatting about the last 10 days, we all exchanged email addresses and the other people always used to write to us in a group email. Unfortunately I don't keep in touch with people very well, if I know I'm probably never going to see them again then I have the silly attitude of what's the point. Not a great attitude to have I must admit. I then left the dinner table to leave for the airport, I felt like a proper jet setter telling my new friends that I was leaving now as I was heading to Thailand. So I said my goodbyes, all the women from the group were in floods of tears and were shaking uncontrollable. They wanted me to stay with them and continue to fill their lives with love and joy. Ok maybe that didn't happen.

Darwin is a surprisingly nice place, I expected it not to be. I walked around the city and it is steeped in history and it was a place where battles were fought in the world wars. I stayed in a fantastic hostel which was in a totally different league compared to Mad Cats in Perth. It even had a sun terrace on the roof with a pool and a DJ.

I headed to Darwin airport in a taxi and arrived at the check in area. I rang home and told my Mum and Dad that I was going to Thailand. I was somewhat intoxicated at this point from my evenings entertaining and I talked some rubbish to the parents.

13. CINNAMON

I arrived in Phuket in the early hours of the morning and got my rucksack and flagged a cab down. I headed to Patong. The air was very humid and it still felt warm even though it was the middle of the night. I arrived on Bangla Road at met up with Martin in The Dream Bar and we had a few bottles of Chang, he had sorted me a scooter which they simply had parked in the middle of the bar. It stayed there for 2 days as I was too pissed to ride it. It was pink and everyone used to call me Ladyboy when I rode it.

I felt great, I was just embarking on a new little adventure and had a good outlook I also had all of the good momentum from the last 2 trip within me. Patong was very interesting, the main strip was covered in bars and the colourful lights were amazing. This time I felt like I had stepped into a different world, the people were so amazing and of course I had only been to countries previously where there are White inhabitants. Martin knew so many people due to the fact he had been there for so many years. The girls were so cheeky and confident and straight away I was having a good laugh with them. The atmosphere on the strip was just buzzing everywhere you looked was just one big party. I had been in Australia for 6 months and of course prior to that my previous 19 years in England and I spoke to more women in one night than I had my entire life. I think it was because they were so upfront it just allowed me to relax and have fun with them.

Of course the girls were only after one thing and one thing only, your money but they did this in the nicest of ways. They are incredibly clever as this is there job. If they don't manage to make you think they actually like you then of course they go hungry. I never thought I would have been persuaded by these beautiful foreign looking women but I succumbed. Its easy to look back on it now and think its wrong but I was a young man who wanted female attention and it was so desperately missing from my life. Of course the day after you hate yourself but you soon find ways to hide the guilt and shame. Then you go and do it all over again.

After about a week all the girls who stood outside the bars and clubs got to know my name and they would all shout me as I walked down the road. I felt like a celebrity and loved every minute of it.

We used to go to this bar down a little side street just of the main strip, it had a pool table in it and some good music. There was this incredibly beautiful girl who worked there and I couldn't take my eyes of her. After a few nights and a lot of beer I got chatting to her and played a few games of pool, I let her win of course. Thai girls are so amazing at pool, it's because when there not working they just sit in the bars playing all day. Over the course of the next 2 weeks me and this girl spent a lot of time together and although it felt strange I just went with it. She was very clever and had about 4 different men sending her money from across the world, I never gave her a penny, just a necklace and my good company.

I'd been in Thailand for a few days and Martin told me about this drug they all smoke which was supposed to be great. I of course wanted to try some Yaba and we got hold of some one night. We went back to my hotel which was about a 5 minute ride on our scooters. We parked them up and headed to my room. Martin pulled out the little package from his jeans and got out these 2 pink pills. We got some tin foil and rolled a bank note up then heated the foil. Martin went first and the first thing I remember about the experience was the smell. The room soon filled with this incredibly sweet smelling scent. Such a lovely smell. I think this is an additive they put into the drug to make it more appealing to kids. I watched Martin suck the fumes that were coming from the tablet. I think he had half and then it was my turn. I was so excited and couldn't wait to try this local drug. Martin took charge of the heating requirements and I concentrated on fume intake. I waited for the smoke to come and I sucked it all up, I chased the smoke around the tin foil making sure every last bit was inhaled. I wanted every drop. I loved it, just like those other times before something happened in my brain and the chemical reaction was just incredible. I just felt so happy, like I wanted to burst. I had this amazing feeling inside and I wanted everyone to know and share the joy. We shared the second pill and jumped on your bikes and headed to the strip. I remember walking into this one bar and the music was playing and I just felt so euphoric. I felt as if everything in my life was just perfect. The drug seemed to last for quite a while, more often than not we would venture out of the hustle and bustle and into the darkness to score some more of the magic pink pill. I was smoking a lot of Yaba and soon the nights were no fun without it. Whist under the influence I was very high and just like before on the crystal meth decided to ring a few people back home. I had a girl in the phone box with me and I rang my Dad who was in Spain at the time, I was saying some extremely silly things and getting the girl to speak to my Dad. The next morning was dreadful and I felt extremely embarrassed and still do to this day. Guess I just wanted him to know I had found myself a girl.

The girl from the bar knew the score and wasn't daft. She could tell when I had been smoking the drug and showed concerns. "Your eyes are crazy Tom" she would say in her broken accent. The girl I was seeing told me that the police do drug tests and if you are even tested positive you get a prison sentence of 1 year even if you hadn't been caught in possession of anything. I had read some extremely good books but also shocking about Thai prisons so I knew full well what the consequences were. The books I read were The Damage Done by Warren Fellows and Welcome to Hell by Colin Martin, they give graphic descriptions of what Thai prisons are like. I was in the process of reading the story of Schapelle Corby and I knew how serious these sorts of places took drugs. Now I became very paranoid at this point and could not get the idea out of my head that I was going to get tested. I had read the Secret and as I was concentrating so much on getting arrested I firmly believed this was going to happen. As the drugs were in my system I could do nothing about it, it was just a waiting game. She told me about this when we were down on the beach. I panicked and didn't know what to do, I said to her that I wanted to leave and head back to the hotel so we got on my scooter. We had rid for about 10 minutes and there was a massive road block and the police were pulling people over in there vehicles. I thought this is it, there going to pull me over and do a drugs test. Luckily the girl knew a different way that took us to the right of the road block and back towards the sea. I shot down there and hoped they hadn't seen me. We then took another turning and found a path that took us along the beach front and back towards where I was staying. I began to hate Thailand and I became more and more paranoid as each day passed. I was convinced the maids in the hotel were planting drugs in my room and I used to come back to the hotel and search it head to foot looking for drugs or any other illegal items. I was starting to go mad. All I thought about was how bad the prisons were over there and that I wouldn't survive. I tried drinking litres of water to flush the drugs out of my system in the hope that I would no longer have any trace of Yaba in my body. I kept a low profile for the remaining few days and just wanted to go back to Australia as it was starting to get to my head. There was so much temptation it was untrue and it was hard to stay away, the girls, the drugs, the drink, that place has it all. I guess that's why they called me Cinnamon.

When I did get out of Patong on my scooter the scenery was amazing, very Green with lovely landscapes the roads were fantastic and windy. I headed to Kata Beach and Karon Beach where there were some amazing hotels. I then came to a lovely harbour and I took a turning of the road and headed to a little market. I was the only Westerner in site and it was so poor. About 15 kids ran along the side of my bike saying 'Hello Hello'. I felt like I had liberated Thailand. From there I went to Promthep Cape which is renowned for sunsets and I wasn't disappointed. There were about 1000 people and lots of little market stalls which was lovely to see. I was just missing something, someone to share it all with. It's alright seeing all these beautiful places but it's rubbish on your own, it's kind of wasted. I did go to Phi Phi where the film The Beach is set but again the weather was poor and I was rather disappointed. I was on the trip on my own and didn't really enjoy the experience. I spent a lot of time with Martin's friends who were all smoking the Yaba, another drug they were taking was Valium which was available over the counter, I decided to try some of this and just went to sleep. One lad, Gorgeous Mel was extremely addicted too it and he was having 30 tablets at least a day maybe more. He could barely even walk or talk. This one day we were sat in the bar having a drink and he wanted to borrow a scooter to get some more Valium so he gets on Martin's bike. He went off on this scooter weaving all over the road. He was absolutely ages and we were getting a bit concerned and wondered what had happened too him. After hours and hour's one of the bar owners rang Martin to inform us that Mel was in hospital. When he came out he showed us the damage, his finger, which had been hanging of was now in a bandage and there were cuts and bits missing all over him. He didn't even realise and I don't think he had felt a thing. He had been to hospital and was covered in bandages and stitches. He couldn't remember a thing. During those 3 weeks in Thailand there were more drugs floating about than a Christmas party at GSK.

Martin had told me that it had never rained badly in August for the 10 years he had been going to Thailand and that if it did then it would last a few minutes and the sun would come back out. Well I think he was telling a few porkies as for the 3 weeks I was there the heavens never stopped pouring. There was the occasional nice afternoon or good evening but on the whole the weather really put a dampener on things.

He also told me when persuading me to go to Thailand about all these amazing islands we would see and James Bond this and Full Moon Party that and it all sounded so amazing yet when I got there he didn't want to do anything or go anywhere. He simply said he had seen it all before and didn't want to do it again. So I was annoyed about that, plus of course the weather didn't help. So I didn't know what to do apart from stay in Patong (for the most part). And that's what I did for 3 weeks. Sit in the same bars with the same people trying to make the experience much better by drinking amongst other things. I mean it wasn't bad but I wanted an adventure, I wanted to see all these amazing places that I had been looking at on the internet before going.

All in all my experience of Thailand wasn't great, the weather was shocking and I mixed with the wrong crowd - I shouldn't have been smoking drugs in a beautiful place like that. It wasn't all bad and the experience developed me as a person I believe.

Thailand messes some peoples heads up that I do know. Every single thing you want from life good and bad is available there but as I keep saying it comes at a cost. And I saw people paying the price. You eat the forbidden fruit and you can expect the consequences. I was playing with fire over there and eventually I was going to get burnt. I did however, like all my life, was building up a bank of bad choices, I had eaten the apple. But what was I supposed to do? Go to work nine while five, no drinking, no drugs, no nothing just a sheer existence. I didn't want that, I would have gone mad which given my eventual fate would have been a blessing. I chose a different course, the road less travelled but one that was much closer to the edge. I'd like to say I was happy with my choices and felt good about myself, the truth was I didn't really and perhaps the nine while five may have been a better option in hindsight. However you have to make mistakes to find that out, no mistakes mean no living, no living means death.

I departed Thailand and was relieved to get away. I still wasn't safe, I still had it in the back on my mind that I was going to get drug tested. I flew via Singapore and in the airport there is a sign which says something like 'we execute drug smugglers' and although I wasn't a drug smuggler I was still worried. I placed my bag on the scales in the check in area and it came up with a figure. The lady then wrote a figure down on a piece of paper which was totally different. I then in my paranoid state believed that they were changing the weight of my bag so that they could fill it with drugs. I tried to tell the check in lady but she didn't understand me and in the end I walked of in a frightened state. I thought this is it, I've concentrated so much on the whole drug/prison debacle that it's coming true. I tried my best to get on all the security cameras, god knows what for. I was clueless as to what to do so I just carried on regardless and proceeded to board the plane. Nothing happened with my bag and I was never stopped. It just goes to show how easy it could be to get into trouble even if you have done nothing wrong and how powerless you are in these places. It also shows how my paranoia was taking over.

I landed back in Darwin and got checked into a good hostel this time after my bad experience with hostels in Perth, it was called Malabooka. My diary states 'I knew I was back in Darwin as the customs man had Khaki shorts on and long white socks, he looked like he had just come out of a wildlife programme'. Some of the hostels are like hotels with great rooms, pools, internet rooms, bars and are generally nice places to be. It was such a good feeling to be back in Australia, it was like I had gone home. After all of the success in Thailand chatting to the girls one night I approached two girls in a take away in Darwin. I went up to them and said something and they kindly asked me to leave as they were having something to eat. The confidence I had built up over those weeks disintegrated in those 10 seconds, I was back to square one once again. I decided I didn't want anymore drugs as it didn't feel right deep down and left me feeling dirty and ashamed. The highs were good at first and the lows were manageable but rapidly the highs became less euphoric and that good feeling I got became all most none existent. Instead you were just left with the lows and they became harder to cope with. The price I was paying became too high and that's when I knew I had to pack it in. If you leave it too late then sometimes you don't have the perception to get out of the loop and you become engulfed. Sadly many people fall into this trap and more often than not the outcome is fatal.

14. LOOK TO THE STARS

I was in a hostel in Darwin and I saw a little scrappy bit of paper with rough edges and a hand written note. It basically said there is a tour from Darwin to Cairns and Cairns was exactly where I wanted to go next. Previous to this I was dossing about in Darwin on my own, after I had walked around the city a few times I was running out of things to do. I didn't really make any friends and was feeling somewhat lonely again. So the advert came at an opportune time. I rang the guy up and it turned out he was new to the touring business and was using this as his first trip in his new truck so it cost very little, it was called 'Savannah Tours'. I remember looking at flights and they were $400. He charged us $300 and there were probably 10 of us. Bearing in mind it was a 10 day trip with all the food and fuel included it was an absolute bargain. There aren't many major touristy attractions between Darwin and Cairns but the scenery is incredible, we stopped and saw a lot of gorges, namely Katherine Gorge. Here a German girl asked me to go canoeing with her which I didn't want too. Of course I did do it and we spent 3 hours out there in the water. It was good actually. There were may other interesting land formations, as Tom the driver was new to the business he was just as interested as we were which made it that bit more special. We stopped in some cracking places and slept in swags which are basically sleeping bags with mosquito nets. The star formations in the outback are out of this world, because we were in the middle of nowhere and there was no other light to dilute the sky, the stars shine tremendously bright, the Milky Way was extremely visible, it was so strong it looked like a cloud in the sky. I used to drift off to sleep looking at the stars and often saw shooting stars, I always made a wish. Whilst I was in Australia I used to gaze up into the night sky, I could often see a star formation which I often used to see back home in England. There were 3 stars all equally spaced apart and shone with the exact same brightness and they reminded me of myself, Alex and Christie. In my darkest, most loneliest times I would gaze upwards and see those three stars and it reminded me of Alex and Christie and I knew when I saw those 3 stars that I wasn't too far from home.

I spent a lot of time with the driver and again there was a mixed bunch of people. This trip was much more like an adventure and we stayed of the beaten track. One night rocked up at this small lake and stayed there for the night, it was idyllic and I loved been in the middle of nowhere. Just like back home when we used to head of walking into the Peak district, I always tended to find some serenity no matter what chaos was going on in my head. I made two friends called Tommy and Eamon who were two backpackers from Sweden. I got on with Tommy the most, he was a fantastic guy and a big Guns and Roses fan, so much so he had a full back tattoo with the Guns and Roses logo on it. I hadn't seen anything Green for such a long time and as we headed closer to Cairns it was such a welcome sight to see something Green. The stark contrast in landscapes is quite something and it's like you are heading into new lands. The tour was great and once again my confidence in meeting new people returned. We arrived in Cairns and got settled into a nice hostel and I went to the same hostel as Tommy and Eamon. Cairns is amazing and such a party place and very geared up for backpackers. There are just bars everywhere and lots of women and I thought maybe I might get lucky and meet a nice Sheila. There was a bar called the Woolshed from memory which used to serve cheap food and everyone used to dance on the tables. Not whilst you were eating I must add, they waited until you had finished. It made such a difference having some. There is a lovely area on the sea front where all the boats were and I often used to sit and day dream about owning my own yacht and how nice it would be to moor up in such beautiful places. There was a German lad called Tobias on the trip from Darwin to Cairns and he was a good kid, he came back to stay in our hostel. I once went out on a night out with him and he didn't buy one drink, instead he used to go round collecting the empties and drank them. He must have saved a fortune over time.

It was whilst I was in Cairns that I decided it would be a good idea to get my eyebrow pierced. I'm not sure what led me to this decision but I went for it. I was drunk at the time and it seemed like a really cool 'traveller' type of thing to do apart from I looked like a dickhead. In all fairness it didn't look too bad. Some people go ski diving however I went eyebrow piercing.

I had about 2 weeks of partying hard but I soon got bored, there's only so much I can do then I need to occupy my time by doing something productive. Plus my funds started to look low, the two trips, Thailand and general living since leaving Perth must have cost me $4,500 so I needed to raise some capital plus of course I had spent significant amounts in Perth.

15. LAVA PLAINS

Tommy and Eamon had got jobs in a place called Innesfail which was south of Cairns and I decided to go with them to try and find work myself. We arrived in Innesfail and it wasn't the most dazzling of places but it was big fruit growing country and all the work was working on fruit farms. I put my name down and within a day or two I was told I could have a start on a banana farm. I worked for an Indian guy and my job was to stand under the bananas while he cut them off the tree with a machete and then I had to load them onto a tractor and trailer. It was hard work, the temperatures were very warm and it was so humid, it was like being in a steam room down the gym. I found myself dripping wet before I had even started. The Indian man would pick me up and drop me off at night, there was me him and his wife all in this Mitsubishi Pick Up and I would fall asleep on the way home because I was so exhausted. He was a decent guy however he used to make me eat my dinner on my own in a corner, I'm not sure why but it didn't really bother me. I stuck it out at the banana farm for 1 week, before I decided it wasn't for me. Tommy met the lady who would later become his wife in Innesfail and they now have a child together. Although I didn't have much money I knew I couldn't stay there and I had to leave. I took the gamble by leaving and I was a little worried my money would run out but I knew I couldn't stay. I went back to Cairns and went looking for work all over the notice boards in the hostels and internet cafes and I managed to get some work for a very wealthy lady who ran a candle factory from her house in the rain forest, this house was the most amazing thing I had ever seen, not only did it not have locks it didn't even have any doors. It was completely open, I quizzed her on the lack of security but she didn't seem too perturbed. The work was basically moving a load of candles into her Lexus to the new candle factory. When I say factory it wasn't like a big industrial carry on it was more of a hobby that was growing in size. Either way it was work and it was very interesting. I also met another cracking kid from Dublin called Nick, we worked together for a few weeks. We hit it of straight away and got on like old friends. In addition to the candle work he also worked in a bar down one of the hostels so I used to go and see him at night and share a few schooners and talk the night away.

The work dried up eventually with the candles so my finance concerns raised there ugly head again. So I was always hanging around hostels trying to find work, and this one time I was in luck.

There was a little note pinned to one of the boards in a hostel advertising for a farm hand. I rang the number and spoke to Steven, we didn't chat much and he asked a few questions mainly did I have a driving licence. I agreed to meet him inland from Cairns by bus. I didn't have any idea where he was but he said the bus would take me to him. I said bye to Nick and left Cairns. I headed towards a place called Mount Garnet which was a couple of hundred miles West from Cairns. The climate at my new location was a much drier type of heat, a big change from the tropical conditions at the banana farm as it was further north, and the landscape had gone from green to red. On the way to the homestead we stopped off and took a diversion up a dusty road to a cattle pen used to sort the cattle. I asked Steven how far off the station we were and he said in his Australian cowboy drawl;

"We've been driving through the station for about 10 kilometres".

Here I met Stan, he was an older guy who was a nice enough chap little on the lazy side. I stood with Stan while he was welding and I just passed stuff and just generally laboured for the afternoon. After that we went back to the homestead where I was to meet Boo who was Steven's wife and Stevie their daughter, they were all very warm and welcoming. My room was like a static caravan and just set away from the house. We used to all eat together in the main house and get showered and sleep in our own digs. I was lucky with my timing in coming to the cattle station as it was mustering season. This basically meant rounding up the entire head of cattle, which was in the region of 7000. These cattle were spread over a 100,000 acre space. Our job was to get the cattle from the field and take them to a station where the calves had their balls removed, ears cut out, an identity tag put in their ear and finally they were branded. Sometimes after removing the testicles we would place them on the furnace used for branding and cook them. They tasted really nice, bit like chicken. The smaller cows where weaned from their parents and put in a separate area. The bulls, if they were still active, were kept in the main section to go back out with the cows. The cows were then sorted and older ones were sent to the meat works and the younger ones were kept to go back out into the field. We used to save some of the calves and not chop their balls off, only the finest calves were selected for this as they would become the future of the business. The owner of the station, Loch, came to help us complete the 3 week muster along with his daughter Lauren and son Alex, they were great kids. Lauren was rather attractive especially in her pink cowboy hat and denim trousers. I thought I could settle for this. It wasn't to be, she had a long term boyfriend, oh well another one bites the dust. We used to have steak for breakfast, cold beef for lunch and more steak for tea. I couldn't believe how much meat we were eating, having a rib eye steak at 6.30am is just crazy. I come from a butchering background where we have a lot of meat but this was just taking it to extremes. My job was to ride a quad bike and sometimes a Honda XRF400 and round the cattle up into a corner of the field, from there we would walk the cattle to the station to go through the process of sorting as I have just explained. There were 3 on horseback, 3 of us on motorbikes and 1 guy in a helicopter. The days were anything up to 15 hours but I was in my element, I was outside riding motorbikes every day, chasing cows and just generally having the time of my life. I met people later on in my travels and they had paid to do a watered down version of what I was doing and I was doing the real thing and getting paid! I remember on my travels from Broom to Cairns seeing the cowboys and thinking wow I'd love to do that, the next thing is I'm doing it. The good old secret techniques were yielding results again. My dreams of rounding cattle from the time I saw them near Darwin came true, I remember we were sat on the bus and we drove past them all. There was dust everywhere and the cowboys were just on there horses looking immensely cool. I wanted to be there. I have since watched the film Australia and I remember thinking I've done a lot of what this film is about. On one of my trips I visited the actual place called Kununurra where the film was set so I related to the film.

One afternoon we decided to do a bit of rodeo, only on smaller cows but it was still a great buzz. Even though they weren't massive they could still kick good. After the 3 week muster had finished Lock and his children and another nice lad called Grant left and it was back to being me, Steven and Stan working on the station. It was Steven's son's wedding and everyone was going including Stan so they left me in charge. I was in charge of 7000 cattle and 100,000 acres of grass land. I asked Steven to leave me a good list of jobs to do. One of the best things I have ever done in my life was leading a mob of cattle to a dam. We had recently put a load of cattle in a new field and we thought they had all found the water but luckily I went back one evening to check and found that about 70 of them were on the field boundary trying to head back to their old field so they could access water. I was on the station on my own at this point. I was on the Honda and had to round up the cattle on my own but they kept trying to get back to the other field. I must have been chasing them for a good 3 hours but I knew if I was to leave them they would never find any water and perish. I managed to get them moving in the right direction, then all of a sudden one would break out and I would have to go back and get it and start again, luckily I am a very persistent person. In the end I got all of them to this dam, it was the most satisfying feeling I've probably ever had, I had saved these 70 or so cows from dying of thirst. I remember just sitting back and watching them drink, I was so proud of myself, I had tried so hard to save them and I had succeeded. I never give myself credit for my successes and always ask myself could I have done more or what can I do next but on this occasion I just enjoyed the moment and gave myself a pat on the back.

Before they went to the wedding Steven told me that the house was haunted. Now I'm not sure if he was saying that to wind me up or it actually was true, either way when it came to being there on my own I was petrified. It was quite a frightening place to be, there were stories of robbers coming and taking hostages then stealing all of the machinery and animals. I was ok in the daytime but at night I was in a right mess, I couldn't sleep, the only thing I could do was drink but my XXXX Gold weren't doing the trick so I would drink Boo's Bacardi just to try and take the edge of.

When Steven got back we did a whole host of jobs and the work was very varied, some days we would drive round the boundary of the fields on quad bikes and check to make sure the fences were ok and if they weren't we would fix them, there was what you call a 'lick run' to complete, this could take hours given the size of the place, lick is an additive to try and make the cows bigger as the land is fairly infertile. I used to listen to John Laws whilst I was out and about on the station, the debates he had on the radio where out of this world and he had an immense talent. It would keep me entertained for hours, I guess he was Queensland's answer to Jeremy Vine. Some nights we would watch a bit of telly in the family house, I am not a big fan of telly I much prefer listening to the radio or music. Some nights I would venture off out on the motorbike and try a find new places, within the station there were 3 inactive volcanoes, it borders with the Undara Volcanic National Park. That's where the station gets it name Lava Plains from I guess, plus there was Lava all over the ground.

I used to ride up to volcanoes and go so far up, then walk the rest of the way. I got a fantastic picture up one of these and it shows the full width of the station, I think the place was about 40 miles wide. It was a fantastic place to live, I probably worked there for 3 months and it was the best 3 months of my life, I was busy in the outdoors and doing things I enjoyed and I loved Steven. The scenery was beautiful and some of the cloud formations early in the mornings were a spectacle in themselves as well as the storm clouds with all the lightening housed within them. It felt like we had stepped back thousands of years. We were self sufficient and lived of off the fat of the land. I managed to save a bit of cash up working there as I had no expenditures, well the nearest shop was 2 hours away so there was nothing to spend my money on plus all my accommodation and food was included. There was however what they called the smallest bar in the world, it was basically a building with a small bar in which sold crates of beer that we used to take back to the homestead. A lot of the people in the bar were workers from the mines or worked on the roads.

After the muster had finished Stephen taught me how to ride a horse, I would have to go out into the fields and round them all up and bring them back to the little field next to the homestead. There was this little paddock built out of thick logs and it looked like something out of the Flintstones. So I put all of horses in this area then I would have to try and walk up to the horse and put the bridal around his neck. I was petrified at first but I became more confident. Once I had the bridal on I could fasten it to the fence. I then put on a rug type of item then the saddle. I then put on my cowboy hat and hopped on the horse. I started of just walking around the paddock very slowly, I didn't dare go any faster. Stephen was in the middle and I was going around him in a circle and he would guide me. I then got into a little trot and attempted to complete a movement known in the horse world as 'rising trot' but I couldn't master it at first. After a few nights of practising in the paddock Stephen let me of into the fields to go roaming. I headed of and it wasn't long before I changed gears into a canter which was much easier as there was no requirement for the raising trot. I let pushed my one horsepower little beauty into 6th and performed a gallop. I was flying all over, lucking there was just miles of open grass land but I had no control whatsoever and my breaking skills needed some improvement. I loved the horse, it was more natural than a motorbike but horses have brains and I believe you never really have total control but I guess neither do you on bikes really when at high speed.

Just before I went travelling Chad got himself caught up with the law for all the wrong reasons. He was convicted of armed robbery although it wasn't as clean cut as that and there is more to the story. But Chad stayed loyal to the end and took full responsibility for the whole event when he could have quite easily received a smaller sentence. Again this just shows the kind of guy he is. I used to write to Chad whilst he was in prison and send pictures, I was very concerned at the time as I thought it would send him crazy seeing me doing all these amazing things and he was locked in a cell in HMP Doncaster however he later told me that it gave him hope. So I was in the absolute middle of nowhere and I would receive letters from Chad. He was extremely comical in them sometimes and would often draw pictures, I remember this one picture he drew was a massive muscle man with a stick man next to it. He'd then put my name next to the stick man and his next to the big guy. I found it amazing how he got stamps for Australia.

One letter read;

I've been training hard so I'm looking sexy as can be. I'll be out in about 5 years so when I do we'll get all the boys together and go on holiday. Are you up for it? I'm gonna try and get a stamp. All my love. X-Commando, Present Convict.

I have more but I can't for the life of me find them. They will turn up at some point.

I decided to buy myself a car for my travels down the east coast, as I was in a different state I could drive again, there was little choice given my location but I needed something reliable given the distance I would be travelling. I went to Mt Garnet and purchased a Nissan Pathfinder from a man named Beagle. He had acquired this name due to his oversized noise which even by my standards was a little large. I think I paid $2000 for it and to me it was a fantastic motor. I remember doing a bit of off-roading back at the station and went up this little hilly bit and got it stuck with the tow bar, I had to rev the balls off it to get it out, that was the last bit of off-roading I did. So now I was all set for my big adventure down to Sydney, I had my cash in the bank and the right car for the job. My first location was Townsville, this was about a 4 hour trip from the station. I said my goodbyes to Stephen and his family, Stevie had even gone to the trouble of making me some CDs for the trip. I was very sad to be leaving, I had found so much happiness at Lava and felt so close to nature, the scenery, the animals and the lifestyle were so far from anything I had ever known and really sparked something inside me that no other place has. All of the regulation and complete utter bollocks of life had been torn away and I was left was a wonderful existence that very few people in the modern Western world get to witness first hand. I think deep down we all want our own little piece of land which we can farm and provide for our dependants. The world has developed in such a way that the true meaning of life has got lost somewhere and the majority of people fall victim to the system, the rat race. It's hard to break away from it, in fact its almost impossible. But for that small amount of time I had. I didn't feel the pressure to mix with a bunch of travellers who I had very little in common with or had any great desire in getting to know. Just like at University where I felt somehow different and alone that feeling was never far away. But on the station I had a use, I was busy and I served a purpose. I could look back after a days work and think today I made a difference. Many jobs I have done before and after have failed to give me such reward. I couldn't stay there forever though as much as part of me did. I wanted to have New Year in Sydney and see the East Coast plus I wanted to leave Lava on a high.

16. CHICKEN TIKKA LUV?

I departed Lava and joined the Kennedy Highway. Although I had mixed emotions about leaving my attention was firmly on the future and my next adventure. Everything was great and then just after driving the Pathfinder for 1 hour I lost my 5th gear - I couldn't believe it. It cost me a fortune in petrol as I only had 4th gear and I was revving the balls off it. Anyway 4 gears were enough for me so I just carried onto Townsville which was another 280 km/h or so. Again I had foolish ideas, my plan was to find 3 girls who wanted a lift to Sydney and out of the 3 hopefully one would like me. Of course this didn't happen, none of my adverts in the hostels attracted any attention so I headed down South on my own. For the record these adverts were commonplace in the backpacker community and often brought travellers together for company and to share costs.   My sheer desperation must have been too apparent in the ad's.   My excitement for my trip diminished considerably once I had reached my first destination. My diary says 'I was having a totally shit day cos my cars a fucking disaster then I walked into my room and met this Irish geezer from Dublin and he had some magic grass and now's very good and who cares if my cars broken and I don't have enough money to mend it'. Obviously not a sober diary entry. All the good feeling I had from the station was replaced by disappointment once I had entered back into the real world. Or the other world depending on your stand point. I was just aimlessly wondering around trying to come up with some plan or idea that would change how I felt.   The answer was simple, all that stood between me and achieving my goals was the simple act of walking up to another person and having a conversation. There was nothing complicated about what was required. I had done some crazy things and been in some tricky situations and survived but the very thought of approaching somebody filled me with absolute fear. Generally speaking in life you get what you put in and when it came to communicating with people I wasn't putting anything in. But for the life of me, I cannot tell you why I have such fears, I guess it's the fear of rejection. Therefore I wasn't yielding any results. By now the realisation was sinking in that I was never actually going to meet any new people and I may be the first person to travel the whole of the East Coast without speaking to one person. I was once again drowning my sorrows with large quantities of alcohol as this was the only thing that I thought made me feel better. I headed down the Bruce Highway and the next place to see was Airlie Beach. This is the home of the stunning Whitsunday Islands. The roads were great and twisted down to the centre of Airlie Beach. It's such an amazing place to see, there are hostels and bars everywhere and it's just full of backpackers. The whole place was buzzing and its one of the places where if I was to move to Australia I would go. Well that's what I thought at the time, it may be different now. Right at the end of the main road it quietened down and there was a market, there were families wandering about and I thought what an amazing place to raise a family.

As always I had made no reservations so I rocked up at a hostel to try and get in, it turned out that not only this hostel was fully booked but they all were. I didn't know what to do and thought I would have to sleep in my car then this woman told me about a guest house down the road and informed me there was a girl who also had nowhere to stay. The girl was German and once again I took it upon myself to make little or no effort in talking to her. I'm not sure why, maybe it's because I'm a complete bell-end. So instead of capitalising on some company and general chit chat I played the 'I'm heading off into town luv catch you later' trick which translates to 'I'm heading of down the road to sit in a bar on my own all night'. I did however make her chicken Tikka Masala but still found no words to say, it was strange cooking for somebody without making any conversation. It was a little like watching Can't Cook Won't Cook with the mute button on. When your confidence is low and you lack that self worth socialising becomes almost impossible. Plus I used to drink even more and at a much greater rate so when I did feel ok enough to communicate I would be so drunk that people would just look at me in disgust and walk away. And who can blame then? I do not enjoy communicating with drunk people unless I too am drunk.

So like the hostels, also booked up were the boat trips that took you around the islands. Whilst I was conducting my 10 minute preparation session before leaving the UK I had looked at pictures on the net of the Whitsundays and knew I had to visit them. My Uncle Mark told me that I needed some sort of plan. He didn't mean I needed a day to day itinerary but just some direction. I however decided that it wasn't an adventure if you had a plan. I wanted to be directed by the events that happened too me. Now in a film that's good but life doesn't always have a Hollywood ending as I was learning for myself.

Luckily I found the last remaining boat trip down Abel Point Marina. I booked on the trip and turned up to the boat with a few crates of the obligatory Tooheys New as did everyone else. The boat 'Pegasus' was a little less luxurious than the others I had seen and somewhat smaller but I boarded the boat, a little nervous of course. It turned out the captain and his girlfriend where originally from Leeds. They were a smashing couple and really added to the whole experience. I had a good few chats with them and they said some nice words to me one night when I was on good form and in good spirits, it was little things like that that kept me going. Although I wasn't creating lasting friendships with the travelling community I had left a last impression with a proper Yorkshire couple which in some ways meant more too me. The boat trip lasted 4 days and there were some great people on board the trip and it was an overwhelming experience. At the end of the trip this Ozzy guy who was a bit of a cock went round all the people in the group asking for their numbers so they could go to his house for New Years in Sydney. I thought that will be great as that's where I wanted to be for New Year. He of course went round everyone but didn't ask me. Sad times. I wouldn't have gone anyway. We did a bit of island hopping and stopped off at Hamilton Island which is where Whitehaven beach is, it was voted the 2nd most beautiful beach in the world and it was truly amazing. But again like I said before its great seeing these places but you need someone special in your life to share them with not just a bunch of wannabe explorers. It doesn't matter where you are or what you are doing in the world happiness can only come from within. It took me well over 10 years to discover this and cost me thousands of pounds however even now knowing all that, when the dark clouds appear my natural reaction is to pack my bags and fuck off. Maybe one day there might be some gold at the end of that rainbow.

I remember one day we went onto this island and there was an Australian lad who liked to inhale a few herbs. He loved the stuff so much that once we were stuck on this island and realising that he had left his supplies on the boat he hired out a jet ski to fetch his gear. The boat was only located a few hundred metres off the beach and he probably could have swam. He didn't even go for a drive on the Jet Ski. That was probably the most expensive joint he ever had! I had a good laugh with the couple from Leeds, there is something about the English sense of humour that other nationalities don't seem to get. One night we all got dressed up in fancy dress using some items on the boat. I went half as a miner and half as a mermaid which attracted some desired attention on the island. The islands we stopped off at were very classy and lovely places, it kind of showed me how the other half live.

When I was in Airlie Beach I went to one of those legal high shops, I'm not sure why I ventured in but for some reason I was drawn in. I had a good scoot about and the memories of my last legal high experience were a distant recollection. I found some slimming tablets that were supposed to give you a bit of a buzz due to them containing a bit of Speed (allegedly). Once I had returned from my sailing trip I checked into a lovely hostel, they were like wood cabins in the trees. I took my newly purchased supply of slimming tablets back to the room and got ready to go out. I took 2 I think before I left the room and went and got a few drinks, nothing much was happening so I took the short walk back to the room and took a few more. I repeated this action numerous times and continued to drink just trying so hard to feel that high. I actually got chatting to 2 English girls and it was going alright considering my inadequacies. By this point I had took about 12 of these tablets and the next thing all of my mouth started watering and I kept going dizzy, I was wired. I tried my best to concentrate and chat with these girls but I was quickly fading and then all something just came over me and I knew I had to leave. I staggered back to the room and got in bed and the whole room was just spinning, I couldn't stop it. I had an immense pain in my head and I knew I was in trouble. I just lay there for hours in this horrific state hoping and praying for the feeling to stop.

17. BEST LAID PLANS

I went and bought another biography from a second hand book shop near the lagoon in Arlie Beach. It was Chris Moyles, I had always listened to his shows in the morning and loved how he and his team all seemed so happy and funny. I would often be in my little prison cell like apartment in Nottingham feeling desperately low and I used to think I want to be like them. I want to feel how they do. I'm not saying these people are desperately happy but they certainly portrayed that to the nation. I read the book in a short space of time in Arlie Beach. Once I had been on the boat trip and been out for a few days I had taken everything out of the area on offer and headed further South in the Pathfinder. I had no guests travelling with me, I had made no friends and still not met any lovely girls, and there was of course the German girl who I failed to even exchange the simplest of pleasantries with. I was starting to get a bit despondent with it all but had a 'must plough on' attitude, I told myself things would change if I just persisted. I headed south and went to Rockhampton next, there wasn't a great deal there from memory and it was just a mid way point. I stopped in a hostel which was practically full of fruit pickers, I didn't stay long here and headed further south to Noosa which is a great town and really grabbed me. It was rather classy place and had a few designer shops, there was a great vibe about it. It was around this time that the song 'The Way I Are' by Timberland came out. It kind of summarised my life at the time in as much as I had no money but felt I still had a lot to offer. Every time I hear that song it takes me back to that club in Noosa. I stayed there for a couple of days then went to Hervey Bay, this was the gateway to Fraser Island. I think Fraser Island is the biggest sand island in the world, it's basically one big campsite with a load of 4x4's travelling around it. You could only get around the island in a 4x4 and that's what we had, there were about 8 of us in this extended Toyota Landcruiser and we all had camping equipment. I think I stayed around 3 days on the tour and met 2 Canadians, a few Europeans and a couple of English girls. One night we were sat out near our tents and I got chatting to this girl. It turned out she was from Sheffield, then it turned out she was from Aston which is where I'm from, then it turned out she was from the same housing estate and lived only a couple of roads away from me. I didn't know her as she was a good 5 or so years older than me but I thought Christ, I must be on for a shag here as it couldn't be any better. But no, it wasn't to be and after the conversation regarding our geographical similarities dried up (5 minutes) she drifted away to talk to somebody far more amusing. However for those short minutes I thought I had found my soul mate. I woke up the next day to witness such an amazing sunrise over the sea plus a dingo had visited our camp and taken a few items for his own personal use. I ended up taking the two English girls from the trip down to Brisbane, we stopped off on the way to Brisbane at a few places and went to the Steve Irwin's Zoo which is an amazing and fantastic tribute to a very special man. A little part of that place stuck with me, if I'm ever in the garden and stumble across a snail that appears lost I don't squash it or throw it next door. No, what I do is I re house the snail in another area more suitable for its habitat. These may not be crocs but I believe every animal deserves a chance and I learnt that from Mr Irwin. By this point the gearbox was well and truly fucked. My guests thought I was incapable of driving. I'd go everywhere about 5,000 rpm and the car would be screaming. Previous to my arrival in Brisbane my fan belt went on the way back from the zoo with all my new guests in. I was just pulled up on the highway thinking I'm not sure how things can get much worse. I tried to obtain travelling friends to occupy my empty seats then once I had filled them the car broke down. I sat there in disbelief and after a couple of minutes of me just thinking what on earth I am I going to do, one of them said 'Tom, what are we going to do?' Like I knew. I'm not sure what we did actually do but we got to Brisbane . I ended up taking the Pathfinder to a scrap yard in Brisbane as 4th and 3rd gears were playing up. It had become a liability, a little bit like its owner. I was well and truly pissed off with my car as I really wanted to drive myself to Sydney in my own vehicle, it had been a dream of mine for some time and it unfortunately wasn't going to be achieved. I think I got a few hundred dollars for my car at the scrap yard, I actually saw the scrap yard on TV back home on a news report which was strange. I checked into a hostel in Brisbane and it was here I met two great people Beth and Claire. Even though they were from the South of England they were actually fantastic company. I really liked Beth but believe it or not she had a boyfriend back home so that was a no no. Still we had a great time and had some good nights out, Beth was the one who got me into cigarettes, she didn't force them on me or anything but she always smoked Marlborough Menthol and after trying one one drunken night I decided to start. It also didn't help that you had to smoke outside in clubs and bars, this was before the UK adopted the smoking ban. So I would go out with some people whilst they had a cigarette, after a while of being stood there I felt I needed something to do and to justify my presence in the smoking area. In the end I started, I remember buying my first cigarettes in a 7-11 in Brisbane, I then realised that I was now a professional smoker. I never really enjoyed smoking a great deal, I felt a lot cooler and it goes without saying that I must have looked a lot cooler. There was a sign on a cigarette machine in the republic nightclub Sheffield that read 'smoking kills but looks cool'. Smoking does kill and must be avoided at all costs but your image improves by 20%. I was probably in Brisbane for a week or so and got to know Beth and Claire very well. We had a lovely time and it was great to meet such lovely people. We often would wonder around Brisbane with a box of goon. Whilst I was in Brisbane I somehow got in contact with Benny and Carol who had a lovely place there looking over the city. I went up to see them and had a great chat with Carol one evening on their balcony whilst Daft Punk played just over the river. I think we both put our differences to one side and moved forward. Benny kindly offered to lend me some money as we had a chat and I explained that I was struggling a little but I declined the offer. I hadn't run out of money but a quick cash flow analysis didn't show an easy ride ahead and insolvency would be inevitable around Christmas. I declined the offer as I didn't really want to borrow my way out however that attitude didn't last. I spoke to my Grandma and without wanting to sound desperate (which I was becoming) I aired my financial concerns and she kindly brought forward my Christmas present as did my parents. I then headed to the Gold Coast and Surfers Paradise. Surfers was great, very cloudy when I was there with the occasional rain shower. Lots of high raised buildings which gave it a modern feel. That sounds like a section from a holiday programme.

18. SAME PATTERN DIFFERENT CITY

I had Christmas Day sat in a bar in Surfers Paradise on my own. It was very overcast which matched my mood. It was quite a sad day because I was on my own and everyone else was at home having Christmas dinner. I thought by this point I would be sharing the day with all my new friends and having a wonderful time. Christmas is a time for being with your friends and family and where I was I had neither. The sense of failure was strong and I dreaded the rest of my life if it was to be like this. I cant really say much more about the day as it was so uneventful and solitary, I most probably have erased the memories from my head. I never allowed myself to get down when I was in Australia but I was in denial and never acknowledged the fact when things weren't panning out how I had wanted them too, I was instead just a man on a mission and wouldn't let anything else get in the way. What choice did I have? I couldn't stop, what was actually the matter with me? I didn't know but I just knew I had to keep on going. On Christmas Day I was watched only Fools and Horses alone in a shitty bar. I should have allowed myself time to rest and take stock of what was happening, I expected to meet loads of people and everything was going to be great but life has its way of chucking spanners in the works. I don't think I was depressed as such, I was just upset, the thing I had going for me was I was always on the move so I would tell myself that things would get better at the next place, I just repeated that attitude all the way around on my trip. But again my old demons were creeping back into my life just like they had done at sixth form, then university (both times) and now in Oz. The truth is they never disappear, sometimes there loud and in my face other days there just very quiet in the background but they never leave you totally. There are those amazing moments when they do but these are rare and I cherish them. The only thing I knew what to do was drink and in hindsight that was probably the worst course of action to take but I was stuck in a cycle.

From Surfers I went to Byron Bay, I hadn't tried surfing yet so decided to give it a go on this day. I had waited nearly a year to go surfing however it turned out the waves were too big and they wouldn't hire out the boards so I never actually got to surf. I can't have been too bothered about surfing otherwise I would have done it before. On the day in question the waves were massive, it was actually the tail end of a cyclone. The waves were as big as houses and it was amazing being in the sea at that time. I got out of the sea about a mile from where I got in due to the current. I've always been fascinated by waves and the power of the sea, so to be in the midst of such a spectacle was quiet something. Byron Bay is a fantastic little place for travellers, there was some great hostels and a fantastic bar called Cheeky Monkeys that is buzzing at night. I got a lift in a people carrier down to Byron with a load of lads from Ireland and we all went out together the night we arrived. By this time my hopes of meeting a girl were slowly fading, my expectations were reduced but I still deep down hoped to meet someone. My approach on that subject was simple, someone will just appear out of thin air.

It was fast approaching the end of the year and I was nowhere near Sydney where I planned to spend New Year's Eve so I got a bus back up to the Gold Coast and then flew from there down to Sydney. As discussed this was not how I had planned to do my trip but for logistical as well as financial reasons plus the forthcoming New Years date I had to come up with an alternative strategy. I met up again with my good friend Tommy from Sweden, as you can imagine all the hostels were booked, the good the bad and the ugly ones. We ended up going to Kings Cross and getting a hostel there. We were very lucky to get anywhere and the hostel itself wasn't too bad but of course the prices were inflated. Tommy, Eamon and I went to the Botanical Gardens for New Year, there was a massive queue to get in, when we approached the front we realised they were taking everyone's drinks off them, I had a big two litre bottle of lemonade with some gin added to it, I had to down the lot. I felt a little tipsy and it was only about 3pm, we got a nice spot and stayed there for a while. The sun was shining and the gardens were lovely. They jut out and look over the harbour, truly amazing.

I found myself a little out on a limb, Tommy was there but he was with some new friends and I wasn't really mixing that well. I ended up drinking a lot that day and spent most of the time on my own aimlessly wondering about trying to find someone or something to make me feel better but unfortunately I never did. I felt down because I was in Sydney at New Year I should be having the best day of my life but instead I felt as lost as I did the night I arrived. As a child I had always seen Sydney on the midnight news at New Year when I would stay up with my Great Gran and have a glass sherry with her to see in the New Year. Ever since then I wanted to go, now I was here I wanted to be back home with all my friends. The trip had had some massive ups and some downs and I guess was a fair representation of life. By now I was on my own and the celebrations started. The New Year fireworks were out of this world, they lit up the whole bridge, boats lit up in the river, all the sky scrapers had fireworks coming from them it was a truly amazing spectacle, and one that gave me tingles on the back of my neck. So there I was, 2008 was here and I was all on my own. I have seen some amazing things in my life, lived some amazing experiences and felt some incredible things but for the most of it I have been alone.

After New Year I was out in Sydney and I felt very lonely, I remember everyone around me was appearing to be having the time of their lives. The way I felt around that time was I was in a gold fish bowl and everyone else was outside of the bowl enjoying life. Although I could see exactly what they were doing I couldn't feel what they feeling. The world I was in was totally different to theirs however in a physical sense we were in exactly the same place.

All the photos and pictures paint a picture that it was an amazing time but the reality was I found it tough. All that glitters isn't Gold (ATGIG).

I did however remember thinking I left Australia a different person to the one that had arrived. Now I'm not sure this is true but I had seen some amazing things, met some amazing people and consumed a large amount of chemicals so taking all that into account something must have changed within me. Also I felt I needed to justify my time travelling and by telling myself I was now a different person maybe someway did this for me. Did I have any mental health problems around this point?

If I had reached a destination in Australia and somebody said this is it then I believe that's when the problems may have arisen as there was nowhere else to run, instead I was constantly running away from something but I wasn't sure what. Maybe everyone struggles with life? Maybe some don't. I question life too much and want too much from it, if I can't accept things the way they are then I do something about it. More often than not my actions don't help and latterly my energy spent on trying to change things has significantly reduced. Some people take out there unhappiness on other people and it's these people that may need the real help however when someone treats you like shit how on earth can you find in within yourself to help them? I don't know either. It appears that certain people don't struggle with anything but maybe they are hiding it. I watched a fantastic documentary about Stephen Fry the other day and it showed him on QI. Anyone from the outside would see that clip and think he was as happy as any other man however he was dying inside and struggling with life. I often mask my problems because you want to show the world you can cope and you're not a failure. Looking back I did need some help but what do you say? Hi I'm Tom I've spent 1 year travelling around the most amazing place in the world that most are not fortunate enough to experience but I feel a little upset as I can't socialise that well with people and often feel a little alone. Then you watch the news and you see such suffering from across the globe whether it be abuse, famine, illness or war and you feel disgraced at yourself for even questioning your blessed life. Consequently you do not ask for help and tell yourself to get a grip.

After New Year I met back up with Claire and Beth and we had a fantastic few more weeks together, a lot of my worries disappeared when I was with them. We went to the Blue Mountains together and visited the Olympic stadium which was a fantastic day trip, we came all the way to Sydney in a boat seeing all the sights plus I was with them which made it even better. We of course had the obligatory Sydney Opera House photos and saw all the sights and went over to the beautiful suburbs over the bridge. Sydney was much older that Perth and had a slight London feel about it. It was a fantastic place to be and part of me wished I had spent more time there. Bondi beach was a little disappointing but Manly beach was much better, I did however apply for a full time gardening job in Bondi boasting my 5 year's experience in weed extraction. I wasn't sure what I was going to do if I got it due to my visa expiring. I had the interview in this guys Ute but he told me I was unsuccessful. I was struggling a lot for cash in Sydney so much so that I had to borrow $400 from Tommy, I gave it him back once I got home. I didn't have a clue what I was going to do, I literally had no cash but I just kept going to the cash machines and praying money would come out of the slot. I never logged onto my account to actually see what money I had, I didn't dare. Instead I just kept hitting 'withdraw'. I didn't know what else to do. I went looking for work and luck would be on my side as I landed myself a fantastic job working with an events management company at Hyde Park, I just went to the office and asked them if they had any jobs, I was passed onto the boss and he gave me a job right there and then. I later found out that he gave me a job just because I'd gone and asked and no one else had done that before. The job was fantastic, I was using my fork lift skills for one of the days working in Hyde Park, just like in the Casino I took control of the operation and helped successfully re locate a large coffee machine (much more complex than it sounds), another day I was sent out to various places in a people carrier to fetch items like tarpaulins and such like, I even managed to drive over Sydney Harbour Bridge. I tried to blag my way over the bridge for free saying I worked for the council and showed them my t shirt but they weren't buying it. Another day this Ozzy lad and I had to go and drop off various items for an event in the Sydney CBD. This one job we had to do was pick up some stuff belonging to a band that neither of us had heard of. They kept banging on about how precious their equipment was and that we shouldn't damage it. We gently loaded the van making sure nothing got broken and neatly loaded all of their tackle, then we slowly and carefully left the road where the hotel was, then my mate floored the accelerator and slammed the breaks on meaning the entire contents of the van went from one end to the other! We had a good chuckle about that.

They even put me up in the Hilton hotel for a couple of nights, I remember there was a massive breakfast laid on and I used to fill my rucksack with pastries to eat later as I had no cash. One other job they had me doing was marshalling and crowd control for 3 weddings (including 1 gay wedding which was new to me) in the street, all part of the Sydney Festival. I took my role very seriously and often said in a cockney accent

"Excuse me luv do you mind stepping back".

I had a nice shirt on with the Sydney Festival logo on it and a list of all the acts on my back, this lovely girl in the crowd asked me for a shirt, I said I'd see what I could do. I ended up going back to the office and getting her a shirt thinking this time I just might get lucky. I gave her the shirt and carried on marshalling as the crowd got a little out of control and they needed me to sort everything out and regain control. I returned back to the spot where the shirt requester had been stood however she had gone. Once again I had been used for my material assets.

Another funny thing that I realised when I was in Australia is that I copy people's accents, for example my friend Tommy had a slight lisp and a Swedish accent so after spending some time with him I started talking with a slight Swedish accent along with a slight lisp. When I was with Nick, who was from Dublin, I started talking with an Irish accent – very strange.

19. HOMEWARD BOUND

Shortly after the festival I booked my flight home. I had no money and to be honest I was ready for home. My visa was about to expire and I had to leave the country. Richard back home lent me a few hundred quid and my Mum and Dad paid for the flight. My flight home was a strange one, it went from Sydney to Tokyo then onto Geneva and finally Manchester. I left Sydney in blazing sunshine and landed in Manchester with my flip flops and shorts on. It was freezing back home in the UK, I landed home in January 2008 and was greeted at the airport by my Dad and brother Alex, it was great to see their faces in the arrivals. It seemed strange at first to be back at home but that didn't last. It was good to see them both after such a long time away. I'm not one for telling stories so kept a lot of my exploits to myself and was fairly reserved. You would expect someone to come home and just sit round the table and tell interesting stories for days on end, I'm not like that, and I take the attitude that why would anybody be interested in what I've got to say. Guess that's why I thought it would be good to write stuff down that way the odd event that may be of interest won't be lost. I remember going down to my local a couple of days after coming home and seeing everybody, I had kept it quiet that I was coming home so all my friends were very surprised to see me. Things were soon back to normal after about 10 minutes and it was like I had never been away. We headed down to Napoleons casino and it appeared all my friends had now become professional gamblers, my mate Adam even used to watch the table and write down all the numbers that came up on a little note pad. He would often inform us that he had cracked the gambling code. It was good to be back with my mates, I felt like I had achieved something and I guess looking back on it now I did. There were many times along the way that I wanted to quit and call it a day but I just kept my head down and carried on trucking. This was probably down to the fact I had exhausted all other avenues left at home.

Me and Richard spoke to each other a lot via email whilst I was away, he always made me chuckle telling me about his own travels in Spain where her worked as a Golf pro. When I returned home our friendship grew, the first place he took me when I got home was a plant hire auction. He was in his element our Rich in this place, walking around telling me all about these special tractors that don't pay road tax. He loves a good sale and fits in very well with the country life. When he took a position in the family business I saw a lot more of him and as he wasn't golfing as much and he was located in Aston.

I wasn't home long after landing back on British soil that I was job hunting, I decided towards the end of my trip that I wanted to become a financial adviser. This was because I wanted to be wealthy and also help people. I believed the 2 goals could be achieved down that career path. So I headed to a financial advising firm on Ecclesall Road in Sheffield, I went into the company just one day after landing and asked if they had any vacancies just like I did back in Sydney with the events management work. This time it didn't work out so well and I was asked to send in my CV and they said they would get back to me but I never heard anything. Luckily for me a good friend of my Mum and Dad's, Richard, managed to secure me an interview at a firm called Westcourt Financial Services. I got an interview with a lovely gentleman called Mike who was the Company Director, the interview went very well and I got a great feel about the place. Their premises were lovely and located near the old snuff mill in Sheffield. It was a great place to be situated. I was delighted to be informed that I had got the job as an Administrator within the firm and I was put on a 4 week probation. I was to deal with contacting insurance companies to chase documents up, send out letters to clients, load plans onto the database, valuations, memo's and general admin related duties. I successfully completed my probation period and Mike informed me that the plan eventually was to progress from Admin into becoming a financial adviser over the next few years. I was expected to complete one exam a year Mike said and I set to work straight away. After one year I had completed all 6 exams and now had my certificate in financial planning and certificate in mortgage planning. They were very pleased with my progress and would often compliment me on my achievements. I probably worked for 1 year in admin then got a job working alongside David who was the Managing Director. David was a very kind man and had a massive amount of respect both within his business and outside of it. Some people have a way about them that people warm too and he is one of these people. My responsibilities increased and so did my work load and I loved it, all I wanted to do was work. I would be in some days at 7.30am when David arrived and would often stay until 6pm. I was learning so much and could see a fantastic future mapped out for me at Westcourt. Over time I built up a good relationship with David who at the time was one of the most successful financial planners in Sheffield. He even put me on the investment committee which of course meant a lot to me. This basically meant going golfing for the day and eating nice food but in all seriousness we did work hard too. I would often make some comment about the Chinese fiscal policy which bared no relevance to the meeting whatsoever and was totally out of context. It did however make me feel somewhat educated. The committee was very important as it affected where people's money was invested and a lot of time and resources were put into the meetings, it made me feel like I had lived out my dream and become a stockbroker. Our funds outperformed many of the benchmarks every quarter and it was great to be apart of something so great. I just loved it. Before I was put on the committee I used to tell David how good I had played at golf at the weekend, then when I turned up I couldn't hit the ball, I used to try so hard to show David how good I was that it backfired on me. They promised me a round at Woodall Spa but after my poor performance they went without me which hurt. So I was in a good place, I had a career which I loved and that meant a lot to me, I had done all my travelling and I was now ready to get my head down. So I was now as my Grandma puts it David's 'protégé'. I got on well with the majority of the staff, it was clicky like all offices and there of course were office politics but I just kept my head down. Karen came back to the company after moving to Australia (not with me but with her family) and I took an instant liking to Karen. We got on extremely well and I really came out of my shell when she arrived. I enjoyed taking the Michael out of her and she certainly held her own. She would also bring me lunch in that she had cooked the night before and I would sometimes return the favour by buying her a Panini. One thing however that I didn't like was the fact that I had to wear a uniform. I didn't know this when I took on the job and I am very picky with what I wear and always want to be smart. So I hated it, one thing I did though was wear very bright socks which were always very in your face and loud, it was my way of rebelling against their corporate image. I even bought similar ties that I wore that looked the same but I knew they were mine.

When I first started I was introduced to Laura, who was by all accounts a stunner. On my interview I was shown into the office and she was there on the photocopier, from that moment my mind was made up. We got on great and Laura was the one who gave me my training (wasn't I a lucky boy) she was married at the time but later separated. There was definitely a spark between us but I was massively shy. I had a good laugh and shared some special times, its amazing how a situation or a place can be changed so much by the presence of a person. After she separated from her partner she moved back home to Grimsby to be with her father. As she was leaving Sheffield she also left Westcourt and of course I was gutted. We went out for her leaving party and it ended up just us two. We had a lovely time and it's a place I often wish I could go back too, just to share those moments. We once went out to town and I met her at her house and we got the tram into Sheffield. She had this White coat on and looked stunning, I remember just walking around town and all the men just used to stare at her. It was a lovely feeling to have such a beautiful women on my arm. She was into her music and she got us tickets to see The Kings of Leon. The whole of their Only By The Night album reminds me of her, some songs especially. We went out for a meal one night and I in my drunken state thought it would be a good idea to set the fire alarm of as we were leaving. Of course I took a mandatory fire extinguisher in our getaway taxi. She was a good laugh and thought it was funny (or at least I think she did?!?)

Laura was a good few years older than me and had a child, we went out for a few months shortly after she left Sheffield. Things were great at first but for some reason I got frightened. I don't really know why, even to this day. I think it just comes down to the fact that the time wasn't right for me. Who knows? I liked the chase and I wanted that feeling of trying to get something to just last. But that is not sustainable of course. Bearing in mind that all I had wanted to do for the last god knows how many years was settle down I now had found somebody and didn't want it. I always want what I can't have and when I get what I want I don't want it. It's like the weather, in the summer I miss winter but when winter arrives I wish it was summer. I suppose being content with what you have is a trait I need to work on but if everyone was content the world would stop spinning. For humans to progress we need people that want more from life, now I don't mean that you should not be content with certain parts at all, in fact quite the contrary.

To be honest I wasn't ready to settle down, I was scared that I was going to have my freedom taken from me, I was still young and didn't want to get tied down which is a contradictive statement I must admit. I didn't treat her with the respect she deserved, I used to get drunk with my friends and be nasty to her. I hate myself for the way I acted, it was unacceptable. I in my deluded mind believed that if I pushed her away a little it would just cool things of and slow things down. Laura was and I'm sure still is an absolute gem and deserved someone who was going to give her the full admiration she warrants, at that point in my life it wasn't me unfortunately. I always tell myself in another life things could have been totally different. I guess I wasn't totally happy with who I was at the time and like a foolish person acted in a way that wasn't true to myself or fair to Laura.

She introduced me to her father and he seemed like a lovely gentleman and had a brilliant moustache, I even went to her house for spaghetti bolognaise which isn't a dish suitable for parent introductions as I had more down my top than anywhere else. In the end she saw sense and decided to end the short relationship and I totally could not blame her. She tried so hard to make it work and in my own way I tried to change my perspective on things at the time but it was to no avail. I still had that part of me that wanted to have loads of girls on the go and to be playing the field. Now I'm a little older I've come to realise that playing the field wasn't my path and wasn't me and if I'm honest isn't probably cracked up to be what I used to think it was. So I was single again after my only real girlfriend since Lucy had left me and with good reason.

20. BACK ON THE GEAR

I went over to visit Nick from Dublin and he took me to all of these old bars in Dublin where the proper Irish drinkers went. We were having a great night and catching up and reminiscing about Cairns. He then says I've got something for us, I didn't have a clue what he meant. The soft lad had only gone and bought a massive chunk of Cocaine, now up to this point in my life I had never tried any of the stuff. Me and all my mates thought only the dickheads down the pub used to fill their nostrils with that shit and by all accounts we were right. But me been me, plus I wasn't on home soil, thought it would be a good idea to try some. I was handed the bag and ventured to the toilet and proceeded to shovel this yellow ish power up my nose using a 1 Euro coin. I had some then straight away had some more and walked back to the bar. I felt like I was 10 men, I just wanted to walk up to everyone and have an extremely lengthy conversation about absolutely nothing. We had a lot of the stuff in a short length of time, my front teeth went numb probably due to the absolute shit that was in it. The coke wore of very quick and I was soon asking my pal for another hit. It was great at first and the Guinness was flowing and we were having a great time, then it wore of and desperation sank in. We had run out and I asked Nick to obtain some more at his earliest possible convenience however he couldn't. All the good feeling left me and I felt stone cold sober. I didn't want to stay out and we went back to the hostel. Despite that night ending in a low we had an amazing time. I was very lucky to meet such a character and spend such quality time with him. That's what life is designed for. Less the white stuff.

I was going out a lot with the lads and I was out drinking every weekend and in great volumes, we had a lot of fun most of the time. I remember once going out with Matt's (my friend from Oz) work colleagues and we all met in a pub in Broomhill called The York and it was around this time that I had an obsession for barking when I was drunk, I just used to go up to random people and bark in their face. On the night where we met all of Matt's friends I just decided to start barking as loud as I could, Kidder loved this and joined in. My mates thought it was funny but most of the people thought I was strange and why wouldn't they? So there you go, I was barking mad. A few of my mates still enjoy a good barking session and on the odd occasion we go through McDonalds drive thru and pretend to have a German Sheppard in the car with us.

When we were growing up we always used to get chucked out from nightclubs and it was said that it wasn't a good night unless we got chucked out, I once got chucked out of a nightclub called Liquid 3 times in one night as I kept jumping over the fence and into the smoking area. We once went on a mad mission in Doncaster and we ended up being chased along the roof terraces of all the bars in Doncaster, I tried hiding underneath a load of boxes but I needed a tiddle so I gave myself in and was met by the local bobbies. I tried to explain to the police that I wasn't a burglar and how could I be dressed like this. He informed me that not all robbers wear black and white stripy tops. My mates who carried on hopping across the roofs got back onto ground level and went in the club, I on the other hand wasn't so lucky. On a separate occasion a group of us went to the cinema to watch Borat and we decided to purchase a few Special Brews, we had a few on the way and took the rest in. The cans just slotted nicely into the drinks holders on the arm rest. So we carried on drinking and left the cinema, I had to watch the film again because I couldn't remember what happened. So we left the cinema down at Centertainment and went into the bowling alley next door. We were messing about as you do and I then told my mate John to get his camera out. I then said a few words into the camera and executed a strike using my body as a bowling ball straight down the middle of the alley. The big machine came down and I managed to free myself and we then promptly exited the venue. But I got a strike.

An historical event took place around this time, the twin cooling towers in Sheffield got blown up and were turned into rubble. These two objects were iconic for the people of Sheffield and were the standard view as you went over the Tinsley viaduct. We were all at a party in Beighton and we were all well oiled. So we headed of down to Meadowhall to watch them fall. There were thousands of people down there. I went down with a friend called Gamby, Gamby wasn't a school friend but a new acquaintance that had joined our club. He is a very wise character and has created significant wealth for himself, he keeps his methods of accumulating such funds to himself. So I headed down there with him in his Black Range Rover. The night was fantastic, Tom who had his tie tied around his head thought it would be a good idea to jump on a roof and dance around like a mad man. Me and Gamby headed off towards the site jumping over the fences and past the guards. Gamby told me if we get a brick each from the towers then they would be worth a fortune. We were gone hours but couldn't manage to get there. We failed to realise the River Don was in our path. But still it was a good night and those towers are greatly missed by the people of Sheffield.

There was a pub called the Wetherby and it was the place to be at one time, it was located on the cross roads in a village called Swallownest. It was where everyone went and it felt like going to a school reunion every week as everyone from school was there. I was in my element, I had an audience and everyone got to know me for doing silly things and I used to revel in it. We used to drink these things called Turbo Diesel's and these were basically half a lager half a cider and a shot of pernod and some blackcurrant. They were deadly, 5 of them and you were on a different planet. The owner Chris went and got a pole fitted in the bar when his wife went on holiday so they could get strippers in. One night I tucked my socks in my trousers and started running and jumping on the pole, it was a great feeling I had all the people in the pub chanting my name which made me just do more stupid stuff. We all have fantastic memories of that place. Fortunately the pub got closed down due to the high numbers of fighting, lads used to come from all over Sheffield to go to the Wetherby that's how good it was. After it closed this meant we could no longer spend all our wages in the pub. Nowhere really ever replaced the Wetherby and by this time it was time we all grew up.

Me and a few mates had a another crazy night in Nottingham as we went to go and see our old friend and the world's number one DJ Armin Van Buren, before we went out we decided it would be a good idea to get the camera rolling again and smash the hotel to pieces. I don't really know why but the place looked like it had been turned upside down and shaken rigorously. Nothing survived and we ended up taking the broken tea cups and tea pot down the next morning in our rucksacks to avoid any suspicion. We even told the receptionist that we were unhappy with the room due to the TV been broke. Anyway we headed off to the club and I decided that I needed to get hold of some chemicals, I spent ages going round all the people asking everyone if they had any stuff. Eventually I got chatting to this one man and he offered me some MDMA. I purchased a bag of these crystals and given the fact that Armin was playing the most incredible music ever the night was just out of this world. For some reason the music just takes me too another level that nothing else does. I got chatting to two girls from Bratislava and I managed to get them back to our smashed up hotel. The lads were chuffed to bits with my 2 little mementos. I did however have to act like we had been broken into when I walked into the room.

Our first lad's holiday was Ibiza, about 15 of us went for 2 weeks and it was pretty mad to say the least. I had a lot of things going of in my head and wasn't really in the best place. It was so hard been in those social situations with all your mates for 2 weeks when your not on your game. I felt like I didn't fit in and that I wasn't very popular. Of course I drank to compensate this and boy did we drink. Me Tom and Matt (Ozzy Matt) were all bonkers on this holiday and caused disruption on a grand scale. Once we came of the strip and there is a fountain at the bottom. Me and Tom thought it would be a good idea to run up to this couple and chuck them in the fountain and run off. I don't think they could quite understand what happened to them. We then ran into a fair and through the dodgems. I lost my chain which my Mum and Dad bought me for my 18th and the next day waking up to discover than was not nice, plus I also lost my mobile so karma was never far away and my theory that your bad deeds will come back to haunt you in some shape or form was ever becoming more substantial, even with such ideas it never stopped me doing such bad actions. So we carried on running and came to a burger king, there was this massive sted head sat eating a burger. Matt then went up to this bloke and poured a super sized cup of Fanta over this bloke. We all then had to scarper.

Ben managed to save the life of a poor dog which was being abused at the hands of its owners. He ran down to some rocks where we were fishing in floods of tears screaming, we all thought he had been robbed. Through the tears he informed us how he fought to free a dog which was hanging from a balcony by its lead. It turned out the dog was trying to commit suicide and Ben had inadvertently saved it.

Tom thought it would be a good idea to go up to a kid in Peppers 2 and tell him that he was a professional boxer. This didn't go down too well and Tom was rushed to hospital for stitches. On one drunken night me and Tom had a little fight, he chucked a bin at me and said 'Big Disrespect'. Our friendship was often put under extreme pressures because if we were both that way out after a belly full of ale we would lock horns and things would happen.

There were riots on this one night and there was a sea of people with a gap in between the two armies, it was like something of Gladiator. During this period Matt decided to go looting and came back to the hotel with the biggest red smile. Not sure what he had been drinking but it most definitely contained something Red in it. There was some altercation between Tom and a bouncer on a separate occasion resulting in the application of Pepper spray, therefore meaning another trip to the hospital. Most of the lads copped of with some women, I of course didn't. We went to all the big clubs and did everything you should do. I was so drunk one night that I decided it was a good idea to eat my ticket for Manumission shortly after we all smashed a coach to pieces, curtains and ash trays were all over the shop. So I had to fork out another 70 Euro for another ticket, how we got out of paying for the coach I will never know. On the whole the trip was good but as I've just said a few darker skies were forming in my world and my extreme behaviour was attracting attention to myself but not in the right way.

Another drunken incident was on a flight to Crete with all the lads, me and Danny started drinking double vodka and cokes however I got a little excited and drank about 5 as I wasn't feeling drunk. Danny who has recently got married, is another good friend I know, he often invites us all up to his stone built cottage for BBQ's in the summer which we all love. He can however drink far more than me but his drinking capabilities are ever decreasing as Big Dave (Danny's Father) will tell you. Dave taught me to drive and I of course passed first time. He apparently said I was one of the most natural drivers he had ever come across in all his 94 years of teaching.

Anyway I then became very rowdy and was approaching all the groups of girls in the departure lounge. Then our flight was called and for some bizarre reason they allowed me to board. Just as the plane was about to take of I started shouting to all the passengers and informed them we would be heading into a 'Lost' type of scenario. I was 100% shocking and all the men were shouting back at me, rightly so as well. I have done some very out of character things whilst been under the influence of drink, something just used to take over my mind and all limitations ceased to exist. It's like I could do whatever I wanted and act or say however I pleased. I was sick on numerous occasions and remember banging my head on the seat in front as we landed which woke me up. I had covered the whole of the back of the plane in my vomit and the passengers looked at me in disgust. I was allowed of the plane, this most probably was down to the excellent work of my friends in calming the situation down. I remember getting of the plane and just sitting near the carousal wheel with my head in my hands going over the last 5 hours. Of course I was deeply ashamed of myself. I was so lucky not to have been arrested, in fact that's what they said was going to happen to me but yet again another lucky escape. That just goes to show how crazy I was after a drink. We had a fantastic holiday in Malia despite my horrendous start. I think I got it all out of my system and didn't feel like I needed to prove anything.

It was around this time that one New Year I made a very stupid promise whilst heavily intoxicated. I promised my friends that if I don't have a girlfriend by the time I'm 30 I will marry an object. I made the deal when I was about 22 so 8 years or so seemed like plenty of time to find myself a woman who I liked enough to call my girlfriend. However now I'm nearer 30 than I am 20 so I'm starting to panic. The problem is what object do I marry and what happens if I meet a girl once I'm married to an object. I will have to get a divorce and it all gets a little complicated. The reason I have added this little bit of information about me is, I don't want people to think in 2 years time that I have genuinely fallen in love with an actual object. It's strange I know but the fact that it's a bet and a joke must somehow make this ceremony more understandable doesn't it?

I went on holiday to Turkey with all my family plus a load of other people as friends of my Mum and Dad's Mick and Caroline were getting married there. I felt very anxious been around all these people and as per usual didn't feel like I was fitting it. But of course I would be able to ease the discomfort and I turned to the drink. One night I was supposed to go back into the town to pick my sister up as it was time for her to come home (she was only 16) however I decided I'd get a drink, then another, then another until I totally forgot what the purpose of my trip to town was. I got in a real mess that night with the drink and ended up lying down near to a sheesh pipe. However I managed to knock over the sheesh pipe and one of the coals fell out and rolled under my foot and as I only had sandals on it burned a hole in my foot. By this point my Dad and his mate Rick had come looking for me, my Dad even thought I was hiding in a toilet and smashed the toilet door down to find a poor Turk having a shit! I managed to get a lift home with 2 Turks on a scooter. God knows how I directed them home, the scooter was going all over with the 3 of us on it. Anyway I got back to where we were staying and got a serious bollocking, and the worst part was they were more upset than mad. I told my parents that I was moving out when I get home as it wasn't fair me being at home and always getting into trouble. By this point I was crying as I was really upset with myself. I was in a mess both mentally and with my foot. I went upstairs and tried to get my passport but they were locked away in the safe. I was going to pack my bags and go home and miss the wedding but as it turned out I couldn't get my passport. I then went to bed after apologising to Rick and Jo for my behaviour. I had been irresponsible in failing to safely return my sister home, having another drink was more important to me at that time. In fact during these years having a drink in my hand provided me with a release and this meant a lot. It represented an exit from any discomfort that was going on in my head. Rather than approaching things and been a man about it I took the easy option. Drink was my medication and with every drink I had it took me closer to the edge. There were endless nights in my early 20's when I didn't have a clue how I got home or I had no recollection of the night's events. This is frightening, the disastrous consequences this could have had are unthinkable.

I woke up the next day and was in a real bad way, I needed medical attention on my foot as the blister was massive, and it was probably 1.5 inches long. I felt shocking, I felt like I had ruined the holiday for everyone. I went to the hospital and got my foot seen too, I had lost my sandals and walked part of the way home in bare feet, and god knows how I didn't do some serious damage to my foot. The wedding went ahead and was great despite the awful feelings I had inside me, my Dad took me and my brother to one side and he was really upset and that made me feel awful, I thought how can I make my Dad feel so upset when he is supposed to be on holiday enjoying himself. The problem was I never learned and I just kept repeating the cycle and couldn't stop, I was addicted to it. I just lived for getting into the pub and drinking as fast as I could. At the time everything else in the world bared little significance, as long as I was in the pub with my mates I believed that was all that mattered.

21. MULTI COLOURED FUNNELS

Whilst I was at Westcourt I needed to earn some extra cash as I had got myself into a mess financially. I had purchased an Audi S3 shortly after starting. I took a £10k loan out to buy the car, at the time my income was £830 per month, once I had bought the car I also bought a KTM EXC 400 enduro bike which cost a lot of money and I financed that by taking out another loan which I couldn't afford. The repayments for the loans were probably £320 and my insurance for the car was £110 or so. So before I knew it half of my income was taken up by my discretionary outgoings. Before I bought the car I never once sat myself down and looked at the figures, I just thought it would be ok and I'll manage. Not even a thought entered my brain that this would be a bad idea. I got the loan and withdrew the money from the bank and headed to Edinburgh with £9k in a bum bag. We and Tom headed up to Scotland on the Megabus and finally a train to the garage. The car was lovely but there was a slight ripple in the paint work on the driver's side door but I was in a tricky situation. I had gone all the way up there with Tom and the plan was to buy the car and travel home. In the end I bought the car. We had a lovely drive down through Scotland and stopped off for the night in Bowness in the Lakes. We had taken all the camping gear and set the tent up right next to Lake Windermere and headed into the town. We had such a fantastic night and there was a great club and Sean Paul's cousin was DJ'ing. We had a right laugh as usual, naturally there was a lot of alcohol consumed. I woke up in the middle of the night with my feet outside of the tent and the rain was bouncing down.

So I had the car, like a lot of things around this time, if I saw it and I wanted it I had to have it. I didn't care of the consequences or repercussions. I think that applied to all aspects of my life at that point. If I was out drinking I had to have as much as I could, if I was going to buy something it had to be something extravagant. I naively believed that such material items would make me happier, they did but like the drink the nice feeling wears of quickly and your left with the mess to clean up the next day, month or even years.

I took an extra grand out to give me a few quid in my pocket after purchasing the car but instead I used the extra cash to get me through a couple of months. Then this ran out and I had nothing else to meet my short fall in income. I then took out a few credit cards to help ease the situation but this of course added to my monthly expenditure. So with the credit cards and other commitments mentioned earlier I had maybe £350 left to survive per month. Then of course there was petrol and the S3 used a lot of oil too, I paid a small amount of board and then of course I needed my beer money and cigarette money. The net result was I wasn't breaking even. At this point with my loan, student loan, credit cards and overdraft I owed £20k. The situation was bad and I needed to do something alongside my day job, so I started working at Aston Hall which is a hotel very close to where I live. I worked there for a couple of weeks as a bar man. This in about 2009/2010 and my car at the time were relatively new and looked really nice. Everyone used to ask me why I had such a nice car and why was doing 2 jobs. The answer was because I was completely stupid with money. I looked a fool, I wanted everyone to believe that I was earning a lot of money and was successful yet behind the scenes I was practically insolvent. I worked there for a short amount of time then due to yet another silly drunken incident I got sacked. One night we had all been out drinking in the locals and I thought it would be a great idea to go up to the hotel with a few pals. Anyway I ended up going up there and causing total carnage, we were in the cellar helping ourselves to the drinks, fire extinguishers were going of and just general foul play. Before I got my job we always used to go to Aston Hall and gatecrash the weddings, Rob used to work there and he would go crazy at us but week on week we would turn up, I remember once Rob greeted us in the reception area with 'Not again'. One night me and Tom had been up to no good in the hotel and the police were called, we managed to get away and headed back to my house through the woods and came out next to our old junior and infant school. The next thing is a police car came screaming down the road and we both set of running. One of the policemen caught Tom but I just kept running. I ran into the school and through the playground and jumped over a massive fence, I slipped and landed on the spike on the top and put a large gash in my thigh totally ripping my G Stars in half. I then limped home. Tom later told me the two policemen had his head against the floor and were trying to force my name out of Tom but Tom never gave in, even despite the threats they made he never gave them my name. So that was another close escape however you can't keep living that kind of lifestyle forever. Lady luck only stays with you for so long.

So I lost my part time job which I needed as it met my shortfall in income. Although it meant working weekends and Sunday and loosing all the time with my friends I didn't have an option, I had got myself into the financial crisis and I knew I had to get out it myself. I didn't know what to do then I saw one of those adverts 'Do you want to earn an extra £400 per month?' and of course I did so I rang the person up on the little advert on my windscreen. It turned out this was Kleeneze. If you haven't heard of it it's basically a pyramid type scheme where you earn commission from selling shit from a catalogue. It sells all household items and to be fair it has some good stuff in it. You make more money by setting people on and having people work under you. You then get a commission for income generated from your own sales plus you also get a lower rate of commission on the sales from any people you set on. You then receive a commission from the people below the people you set on and on and on it goes. In theory as each layer is added you get richer. Say you set on 2 people who set on 2 people you have 6 people working for you. If those 2 people set on 2 people then you would have 14 people working for you. There was the potential to earn a lot of cash, some people at the top were earning mega amounts of money and I was very hopeful of making a good wage from it. I believed I could get people working for me and that things would progress. You have to pay for the magazines and there is a lot of work involved and the money is poor at first. I even went along to a Kleeneze conference which was a great experience. There were a lot of inspirational speakers and I learnt a lot about networking. One man had earned a lot of cash from the scheme and did a talk, it really got me thinking. One thing they did was promote the idea of visualising your goals, for example when I went round to the house of the people who set me on they had pictures of nice cars and fancy holidays on their fridge. This was kind of what the Secret told me. I'm not sure how they finished up but I'd be interested to know how the people are doing and whether the concept of visualising your dreams helped them achieve any of theirs. In the end I lost the drive for the scheme and gave it up as a bad job, I think I just about recouped my set up costs and given all the hard work I put in I made almost no cash. I would be out until 10pm at night after work dropping of or picking up leaflets, I'd then input which houses made a purchase and which houses returned the catalogue and which ones told me to leave them alone on a spreadsheet. I'd then have to make all the orders, deliver the orders and collect the cash. I remember driving about 3 miles to someone's house to deliver 3 funnels which I sold for £2.50 of which I probably got 10%. She didn't even answer the door, I've still got those multi coloured funnels in the garage and everytime I see them it takes me back to the Kleeneze days.

I had a few meetings with the people at Westcourt and tried to show that by completing the exams and taking on a much more involved role I would need financially rewarding. In the end I was given a considerable pay rise which eased my concerns slightly and meant I broke even each month without having to work part time. I sold the S3 after 6 months and bought a Corsa van, now don't ask me how I came to such a decision as I will never know. The van was the most useless van I had ever seen, I couldn't even fit my lawn mower in the back and I had to strap the boot down. I had more space in my polo. People must have thought I was bizarre, I was training to be a financial advisor driving a Corsa van. I sold the S3 for £8k to a lad in Gleedless, I put the money in the bank. I planned to pay part of the outstanding loan with the proceeds from the sale however the bank wouldn't let me do this and said it had to be the full amount. So in the end I made another silly purchase and went and bought a 25th Anniversary Golf. I even bought the car in total darkness in the rain again with Tom. Who in their right mind buys a car on a winter's night when you can't see a thing. Well I guess I wasn't exactly in my right mind. The car was ok actually and I got away with it.

22. SPEED OVERDOSE (PART II)

I stayed of the class A's, well pretty much anyway. Had a few crazy nights out on the white magic, one night I had been at a party until about 5am. When I got home I couldn't settle or rest so I thought it would be an opportune time to go and cut the grass at the Yellow Lion. So I put my earphones on and off I went. Well the job normally took an hour but on this occasion it probably took 30 minutes. I was absolutely flying and my stripes where straighter than ever. But apart from those few instances I just stuck to the drink.

Me and Kidder had a great time on our enduro motorbikes, we went touring round the peak district and on one trip even managed to ride in Yorkshire, Derbyshire and Staffordshire. We went to a place called Three Shires. We used to ride with a club called the Trail Riders Fellowship and the blokes in that club were fantastic. One person was a man called Fred, he was roughly 75 and still rode with everyone all day. Fred would move the earth for you and was very helpful. He was a great bloke but sadly he died this year. It was such a shock to hear the news and a great loss. He had a massive convoy at his funeral and that goes someway in quantifying how well liked Fred was. It just shows that age is just a number and doesn't stop you living your dreams. Until his last days he was doing exactly what he wanted to do and that must have given him a great deal of satisfaction and you could tell when you spoke to him.

The scenery we saw in the Peaks was amazing, we would ride through rivers, up the side of massive rock edges and generally anywhere we saw fit. As we were in the club they knew all the legal lanes to go one and of course we would occasionally slip in a cheeky public footpath just to annoy the ramblers. Kidder used to plot the routes on his phone so we could go out on our own. Kidder used to ride moto x as a child and his skills have never left him. There is this one lane which you fly up a long windy lane and it goes on forever, eventually you get to the top, it opens up and you look out over all of Derbyshire. The view is amazing and never fails to disappoint me. If we weren't in the Peaks on our motor bikes we would be finding some lanes on our push bikes or walking. The Peak District is our playground and I feel at home out there. I recently got back from Wales on my motorbike and we came back through the Peaks and although Wales was good it wasn't ours.

I also had some good days out with Stuart who is my Uncle Mark's mate, he was a great person to go out with and is a very infectious character as well as a renowned businessman. One night me and Kidder went out into Conisborough quarry along with Russell and the other blokes from the club, went deep into the quarry and were flying around for ages, we then found this lovely little pub and had a pint. We all then headed through this wood in the complete darkness and got totally lost, we were stumbling all over the place in fits of giggles. Some nights we would head into Clumber Park and head out towards Nottingham, all of road. Russell told me once that if I wanted to come out with him again I would have to get a new exhaust as mine was too loud and people would complain about us. Of course I didn't but my bike sounded awesome. Me and Kid once got in a bit of trouble on our bikes, we went through the village and came up behind a police car, the police car then pulled into the side road near the fire station and we both went past him. At this point half of my number plate was missing after I had fallen of but decided it would be a good idea not to replace it for obvious reasons. So we rode past a police car and for some reason we then floored our bikes as we headed up the bypass, I turned my head around to find the police car chasing us with his lights flashing, I shouted to Kidder that we had to lose him so we continued to try and get away from the police car. The adrenaline was pumping at this point as I knew we might be in trouble. We then pulled up in a small housing estate and we thought we'd lost him, we were there for a minute or two then this police car with the lights on stormed down the road after us, luckily I saw him and we sped off again. We headed out of the little housing area and down the road and then went off road and lost him again. We waited in a field for a good 20 minutes and I was convinced they were going to get the helicopter out for us, plus a helicopter flew past us. I told Kidder not to use his phone as they might be listening to us and could track our location, that was my paranoia taking over. We eventually carefully and slowly made our way home, we expected to be greeted by the police when we got home. We didn't though. We had got away again. I had escaped again but the ice I was standing on was becoming thinner and cracks were starting to show. My life was becoming more and more out of control.

It was around this time that me and Kidder spent most of our time together and we became very close friends. Kidder is a very likeable character and good fun, we had some great times during that time. He was single and so was I and it was at a time when most of our other friends had girlfriends so we would always be out together getting into trouble. I have been very blessed along the way with good friends. We used to go out and drink power rounds, these were a pint of beer and 2 double vodka red bulls. It was around this time that we used to spend a lot of time in the Yellow Lion which was our local. That's how I got the grass cutting job, it seemed a good idea when I was drunk. I remember been so happy in the pub, I remember thinking to myself I would be happy if I just came in here all weekend and drank 15 pints of John Smiths every night and did nothing else with my life, no holidays no nothing. All I wanted to be doing was to be out with my mates drinking. Its crazy how life's perspectives change. I'm not sure now if I was truly happy at that point, it felt like I was at the time and I couldn't have really asked for anything else from life. I felt I had become the person I wanted to be, as I was out a lot I would always be acting the clown and trying to make people laugh. At the time it really felt like I was genuinely happy. As I've said earlier being out drinking with my pals was the most important aspect of my life. Could this happiness and carefree existence last?

In addition to seeing a lot of Kidder my other closest mate was Richard, we used to go out for a couple of pints on a Monday and end up staying all night eating scampi fries for tea. Richard's Dad would always ring him up and say when are you coming home for tea as it was in the oven. He'd never have his tea, much to his Dad's delight. We used to ponder about the world and put our slant on things, most of the time there was only us in the pub as it was mid week. We would get into very deep conversations about the world, Rich is a deep thinker like myself but seems to be able to channel this in a much more constructive way. I tend to just keep going around in circles thinking about the same thing over and over again and never make progress. He's a true friend is Richard and is much wiser in certain ways than me and we would always evaluate each others latest business idea. He too eventually split up with his girlfriend and in the summer of 2010 we did a lot together including playing golf and single handily kept the John Smith brewery in business not to mention Scampi Fries and the Yellow Lion. I would often go up to the stables to see him for a coffee, he started out right at the bottom in the business and slowly worked his way up. He is now a significant asset to the family business. It's probably down to him being such close mates with a trainee financial advisor who came close to bankruptcy before reaching 21. He's our village equivalent of Del Boy and he is always selling something. He's got a good eye for a deal and can always make a profit, he's given me a lot of advice on that subject however I just don't seem to have the head for sales. I guess you eventually find your purpose in life. So I had a lot going for me in theory and felt I was heading in the right direction.

23. THE PERFECT STORM

I wasn't seeing Tom much or having a great deal of contact with him around this time, I selfishly found this saddening as we had spent so much time growing up together and created so many fantastic memories. It seemed like I had gone from speaking to him practically everyday to almost nothing over night. I would always want to pick the phone up and give him a call for a chat but I stubbornly didn't and took the attitude that if he isn't going to bother ringing me then I wont ring him and we kind of entered a stale mate situation. The truth is I probably needed to talk to Tom more than he did me. Me and Tom had gone in separate directions, he had settled down in a serious relationship and I still acted like I was 17. I also expected Tom to want to do the same. In reality Tom had grown up like most normal people and had seen a better side of life that didn't involve spending all weekend sat inside the same four walls drinking his way into oblivion. Its one of my many weaknesses, I expect too much from people and take things personally when people don't make stay in touch or ring as often. The truth is friends grow apart and this is normal but for whatever reason I couldn't grasp than concept around this point in my life It's something I really need to work on because being reliant upon external factors i.e. peoples actions is not a good way to live. People will always let you down and more often than not you are left feeling crushed and hurt. I try my best these days to kind of let things slide a little but I do find it really difficult.

I had been working with David at Westcourt for about 6 months and things started to not feel right. These bad feelings within me seemed to take over very quickly but I guess it reality they were more gradual than I remember. If you rewind a short time period back everything seemed to be going great however now the years have passed and I have had chance to reflect and think about my true feelings deep down and maybe I wasn't entirely happy, instead I was just trying so hard to live life to the full that I even convinced myself I was happy. I so badly wanted to become a financial adviser but I had ambitions like becoming the best adviser in Sheffield. I must have thought that by achieving such goals I would feel happier within myself. I have always thought and people have told me, aim for the stars and that's what I always did. I never had a practical ambition. What I should have thought was just get a few years experience working with David and then move onto actually selling financial products but I of course wanted it all and I wanted it now. I didn't feel respected at this time and felt that by achieving certain things or become wealthy I would receive such respect. It was around this point that I lost my life compass and my overall wellness started to decline. I was in a bad situation financially which didn't help, the hangover from my spending had kicked in. The bad feeling you are left with when you spend money you don't have lasts a far greater amount of time than the enjoyment you derive from your purchase. I just couldn't seem to take control of my finances, I would log into my bank accounts and just stare at the figures not knowing what I was going to do. I had tried earning extra cash, increased my income but things didn't really improve. Earning a few hundred quid a month extra is a drop in the ocean when you have, what to me, was a large debt. Plus the more money I had the more I went out. I was becoming increasingly unhappy with who I was, I would look at myself in the mirror in a morning and just hate the reflection. Then when I spoke I disliked every word that came out of my mouth. Eventually I criticised every action I took and things got worse and worse. I would hate having to make conversation with people and would avoid situations where I would have to speak. At this point I just withdrew myself from the world and I began to slowly sink below the water, I wasn't under yet and still grasped for the ever declining oxygen.

Although I was already having a lot to drink I began to drink even more. Previously the drink turned me into a different person, a much more comical or entertaining person but when my mental health had started to deteriorate alcohol no longer gave me the temporary lift I used to get. My main weapon in dealing with the negative feelings within me had been taken away and I was now unarmed. This didn't stop me drinking, instead I just used to drink much stronger drinks and in my case Vodka. I would drink Vodka when I was 'alright' just to get more drunk but now I was drinking the stuff out of sheer desperation just hoping that with each glass bottom I emptied there would be some answer or way out. Of course nothing positive came out of these binges, I would often be on my own in the pub not even with company. This of course meant my financial situation deteriorated even more. I didn't really have any problems or a reason to be in such a depressed state. Well not one that I felt was justified for how I felt. I had excellent physical health, a good job, loving family and many friends. But that unfortunately is insignificant when it comes to depression. I could have been earning £50k, married to a beautiful wife and have a holiday home in Monaco but I would have still felt exactly the same. If anything I may have felt even worse because I had so much and still didn't feel right, I possibly would feel a lot of guilt for not being grateful with the good things I had. I was disgusted with myself. This of course fed into the already very negative thinking cycles. I said to myself everyday 'what is wrong with me?' I questioned every thought in my brain and the conclusion was never anything that made me even the slightest bit better. I was still functioning very well at this point and I don't think anybody thought there were any problems. My Mum had questioned me a bit about going out so much but nothing that hinted she suspected I was not right in myself. I was still going to work but there was this Grey cloud that had formed over my head, it wasn't anything major but a storm was brewing.

Around this time I was doing a lot more technical work and was getting more involved with the financial planning side of things and started to influence where money was getting invested. I had got to a point in my career where up until now I was very happy and I got a lot of job satisfaction plus I got the impression that David was happy with my efforts which was very important too me. I remember going out for my first client meeting with David and this to me was the pinnacle of my career since I started at Westcourt. Up until then all I wanted to do was to go out with David and see clients. It just so happened that around the time this opportunity was gifted to me my head was in a real mess. Prior to this meeting my confidence levels were practically on the floor and all I wanted to be was alone. Everything went from bad to worse, I remember my electric window breaking on my car going down the M1 on the way to this meeting which meant the window was fully down, then I got lost and parked in the wrong place meaning David had to come down the road to find me. I just wanted the ground to open up a swallow me up. Then of course David saw my window was down so I explained it had broken and things just spiralled out of control. The meeting at Maltby went ahead, a little later than scheduled due to the technical difficulties. I remember sitting there in absolute owe of David, he knew so much and could answer any of their questions with such speed and knowledge. All I kept thinking was I will never be as good as him and that I can't do the job. I always used to tell myself that everything will be ok when I get out of the office and become an adviser, this meeting was a reality shock as it showed me just how far I was from my dream. I felt like a spare part throughout the meeting and didn't have anything to say, I felt like I had let David down. As my depression worsened by the day so did my intrusive thoughts. Intrusive thoughts are involuntary thoughts that enter into your head and cause distress, when your mental health isn't too bad you just brush off the thought and don't think anymore about it but when you are unwell you pay attention to it and analyse it. The thoughts are more often than not extremely unpleasant and in my case the thoughts are the worst possible thing I could think of. Its like my mind tortures me, it knows exactly what I don't want to think and then projects that thought right to the centre point of my brain. For instance I had a thought to go over and punch one of the clients plus other more bizarre thoughts. It's very hard to talk about what goes on in my mind especially if you don't have any prior understanding of intrusive thoughts. I have since talked about them with various professionals and have felt much more 'normal' about the strange thoughts that exist within my head.

After the meeting I analysed what had happened and of course the thoughts I had throughout the meeting were at the forefront of my concerns. I thought crikey I'm a really bad person for thinking such horrible things, why am I thinking that? Again these negative feelings fed into the horrible sinking feeling that had now took up permanent residency inside my stomach. When I got to the office the next day all the girls in the office were asking me how it went and I tried my best to be talkative but my concentration levels were slowly fading and keeping up conversation was becoming more difficult.

Shortly after that meeting I went away golfing to a place called Mottram Hall which is located in a lovely part of Cheshire, this was a 2 day event and one that I had organised and about 20 lads attended. It was around this time that I had started not sleeping. Up until this point I was still sleeping, I was waking up earlier and earlier in the mornings but would still manage to get a few hours in.

It was around the time of the golfing trip when I first started noticing myself that things weren't ok, things weren't right far before then but it kind of became normal and I just kept battling on however when I was away I remember being on the golf course and I was going through all of my options and this time I couldn't come up with a solution which in the past has been to move on. This time however I decided to myself that I was going to give up. This was the first time in my life that I had accepted defeat. I couldn't run away, I had no money, I had massive overheads that needed paying. I now was frightened as I knew what would unfold before me would be horrific. I didn't want to work, I didn't want to communicate I just wanted to be alone. I had mapped out the consequences of my decision to give up and they were bad, very bad. I would probably go bankrupt, my family and friends would think I was the biggest dickhead known to man. I thought I was the biggest dickhead known to man anyway. I knew nobody would understand what was unfolding in my brain and I suddenly felt detached from my loved ones and knew that the storm was getting bigger and that this was no normal storm this was in fact the perfect storm.

Every element of my life was now crumbling before me, each day a small fragment of light within me was extinguished and one by one the shutters came down. I just had no more fight left in me, I was empty. I had tried so hard for all the years to fight the inevitable, it often felt like I had succeeded but my flood defences were no longer high enough and the tidal wave finally engulfed me. I hadn't done bad really, I had been fighting this moment for a good few years, others would have fallen a long time ago but my time had come and the party was over.

I couldn't pin point exactly what was wrong but it was just an overwhelming feel of loneliness, fear, guilt and darkness. When I caught a glimpse of my reflection all I could see was an ugly person starring back, I was disgusted with the image I saw. I would be extremely sensitive to criticism and if someone said even the slightest bad thing to me then I would feel crushed. Obviously a weekend away drinking with the lads didn't involve a lot of niceties and there was of course banter to deal with. My Dad's friend one night said to me

"You know you Tom, your very needy"

Normally I'd think shut up you soft twat but on this occasion I took it bad. Richard was away this weekend and I felt like I was rubbish company, I didn't have any spark or humour in me and thought that Richard would much rather be spending his time with other people. Me and Richard spoke after a few beers and I opened up to him telling him about the meeting with David and how I realised I was not good enough. He was very supportive and said some kind words but people's words were no longer enough. I'm not sure exactly what people thought was up with me, if they thought anything at all. Maybe people just thought Tom's been a bit quite or a little off with people. I played so bad at golf, I didn't want to be there whatsoever and was just in a trance. I even played the wrong ball on a few occasions which caused a few problems. Luckily Josh rectified the situation. When it came to the end and adding the scores up my brain could not function. I just couldn't add up, my mind was slowly closing down and simple tasks were now becoming hard. On the second day I was rushing to get on the tee and couldn't find my shoes, so I panicked I didn't know what to do. I didn't want to embarrass myself my saying I had lost my shoes so what I did was put someone else's on. This of course raised some questions when the bloke was asking where his shoes where, I was the only person there. I naturally replied 'I don't know' and he then said 'well you've got them on'. That just exemplifies how bad I was becoming, I just didn't know how to make decisions. When we got back to the pub at home after the golf my Dad asked if I wanted to get some tea in the pub or go home. I just couldn't answer, its hard to explain but I simply could not use any sense or reasoning and make a choice. It was like he had asked me a question about a topic I knew nothing about. I had lost a part of my brain which allowed me to process information. I simply could not reply, I tried so hard to think which place I would prefer to go but there was nothing. This lack of judgement and decision making abilities deteriorated further and soon the simplest of questions seemed like words from a foreign land. Day by day my brain was shutting down, each day my situation got worse. I still wasn't sleeping, it felt like my safety cord had been disconnected and I was now floating into the depths of outer space alone. All I could see ahead was darkness, no life, no nothing.

I remember going out after the golfing trip Thursday, Friday, Saturday and Sunday night. I was mostly on my own but sometimes with a few people from the pub. The summer prior to my depression me and Kidder were hanging around with a couple of girls from the pub and we used to have a good laugh. We would get drunk and all have a good time, however on this occasion when I was out with them I was in no mood for jokes. I was just knocking the drinks back and failed to show any signs of fun. I just used to smile a lot and laugh when I felt I should this way avoiding any suspicion that there was anything up with me. We headed of into town on the Sunday night, don't have a clue why but when we got there we ended up coming straight home. One of the girls left her handbag in the taxi so I ran after it and fell over, ripping my jeans and scuffed my shoes. So we got another taxi and went home. It was a disastrous night by all accounts. Previous to Sunday I had felt very bad in the mornings after drinking the previous night but once I got home from work I just started to drink again to try and take away all of the bad feelings floating around within me. Then of course Monday came round and hit me like a sledge hammer. I had the hangover from hell and all my problems came back to me but this time they were worse. Prevention is better than the cure, well that's what my mechanic friend James says when talking about my car. Its true in life, if you just keep on plastering over the cracks eventually they come back but when they do major structural work is required. My Mum came into my room on that Monday and said

'Tom you need to go to work'

To which I replied

'Mum, I cant I'm too tired'.

Obviously like everyone else, my Mum had no idea what was going of in my head or the fact that I hadn't slept for a considerable amount of time. In the end she told me that I must go to work and of course said I needed to stop going out so much drinking. I had to physically drag myself out of bed, this awful fear had set in now, its hard to describe how it felt but this sense or dread hung over me. It's kind of like you know something really bad is going to happen but you don't know when and you don't know what. I got to work that morning and had a pile of work to go through, previous to my difficulties I used to love coming to work and having loads of work to do. This morning I didn't have the same enthusiasm. I just sat down at my desk and starred at my screen. What on earth was I going to do? I was incapable of functioning at a basic level, all I could do was breath. I didn't want to eat, I could not speak very easily and my words were very jumbled up. I would forgot what I was saying mid sentence and in the end I just didn't attempt to talk. I would go out at lunchtimes and just walk up and down Ecclesaw Road hoping to find some answers or solutions to this situation that I had found myself in. After sitting at my desk for what seemed like hours I suddenly got up and walked out of the office and when downstairs to another little office and just sat there. Someone must have rang Jane who was the office manager and on the top floor. She came down and I started talking to her, I was saying all these random things that I thought were wrong with me, I cant remember many but one thing I said was, when were all in a circle talking I never have anything to say and don't feel part of the group. Of all things to say I said that, but that just proves how bizarre this illness is, it was just little things that had built up. It wasn't just things like that, it was a much greater problem but I simply couldn't say what it was. Jane is a very wise person and said some kind words. Once she had left the office she rang David as she probably didn't know what to do. After all her vocation was office management and not psychiatric nursing. Jane put me through to David and it was great speaking to him, he assured me that there were no problems at work and that I should not worry. He said he often gets stressed and I will always remember this, he said

'No problems are insurmountable'.

Initially I felt a lot better but soon that nicer feeling faded and the cloud descended upon me again. Nobody knew how poorly I was, if I'd been this physically poorly I would now be on a life support machine in intensive care at the Hallamshire. I had been down before and felt lost and alone but this was something else, this was terrifying. This time there was no way out, I could not see a solution. I had used up all my lifelines, the phone a friend option had expired and the question didn't make sense. I needed to get away but there was nowhere left to run. As it dawned on me that there was no way out and that the problems inside my head were too big and unfixable I was left with one final way out. The only solution to rid myself of this pain deep within my soul would be suicide. On the walks at lunchtime I would often want to jump in front of a passing vehicle however the road wasn't very fast and I concluded that such an act would not be fatal. My feelings got worse and I became more desperate for an end. I googled various suicide methods and there is some shocking information online plus a lot of people in need of serious help out there. I had considered hanging myself using a towing rope but felt the pain of death would have been too much and not quick enough. I wanted something quick with the least pain as possible, the next method I considered was going down to the railway tracks in Sheffield and jumping in front of a train. What I really wanted was a pill, I wanted to take a pill and just go to sleep and never wake up. If somebody would have offered me that option I would have taken it without a second thought. I don't think I have put into words how dreadful I felt, there are no words in the dictionary which describe how I felt. The only way for you to truly feel how I felt inside would have been for you to be put inside my head. That way you could feel for yourself the suffering and torment that was going on in my mind. I regard myself as a very selfless person and I always consider the feelings of my closest family and friends close to my heart. The act of suicide is regarded by many as a selfish act to take because after all in theory the person who commits suicide then leaves everyone else around them in pieces. However I wonder who would want to continue with there life when their mind has become so poorly. If your mind had a window and people could see inside it and there was some way in quantifying or showing to the world how you feel then I truly believe people may be a little more understanding as to why people decide to make the ultimate choice. It's only because I have felt that pain inside that I can understand the subject more. I guess if I hadn't then maybe my view would be less understanding however I still feel I would show more compassion than some of the narrow minded idiots I have had the misfortune of sharing conversation with.

I didn't put any of my plans into force however suicide still remained the only option and the only answer. My physical presence was still in this world but my spirit had now gone. My parents had noticed my behaviour had become different and my Mum had tried to get me to talk to this man she knew who was a dietician but also a psychologist. I didn't want to talk to anybody, I was frightened about telling people how I felt inside as the things floating around upstairs were so disturbed. I had googled information about being sectioned and read that it was an horrendous experience and that these people were never right again plus of course I was worried about the drugs they administer. Up until this point I knew very little about psychiatric hospitals or sections but for some reason I knew that that very frightening prospect may be forced upon me. I refused to speak to this person my Mum knew, my Mum was a bit upset that I wouldn't accept help. After more persuading and due to the fact I had very little fight left in me I agreed to talk to him. My Mum was pleased about this, my Mum got me a glass of water and I went to my room to ring this stranger. As soon as he answered I became extremely paranoid, he was talking about all these things and it meant very little to me and I couldn't concentrate. I panicked and made the assumption that this man was working for the FBI or the police, he kept asking me these searching questions and I thought he was trying to stitch me up. I knew the things going of in my head were really bad and that if anyone found out what exactly was going on then I would be thrown in a prison cell and never let out. I began to pace up and down my room, I looked out of my room and the family across the road were outside which was a little unusual. The son was reversing his car and parking it so it was facing down the road. I thought to myself why is he doing that, he never does that. I believed he was parking his car that way so he could quickly get in his car and chase me. I now thought that not only was this man on the phone working against me but all of the neighbours and worst of all my own mother. I didn't want to talk to this man and I had to get out of the house, I thought that this was the moment when I would be taken away. I ran out of the house and got in my car and drove to a mans house called Stuart who's grass I used to cut. Nobody followed me. I thought that maybe they had left it for now but would soon come and I would be taken away then. When I arrived at Stuart's my head was obviously in a real mess. The plot was unravelling and the extent of my troubles stepped up to another level. I got out of the car and walked over to get the lawnmower and Stuart came out. I couldn't really speak at this point and my pending fate was all that was on my mind. He came over to me and informed me that his wife had sadly died. She had been poorly for sometime but the news was an incredible shock. I didn't know how to react to the news, I wouldn't have known in a normal state of mind but this really put my head in a spin. Stuart is a great person and I wanted to say something constructive and nice I guess. Stuart and his family were on their way out and he wanted me to cut the grass, so I did. My fears were now becoming far greater and I couldn't take much more on board. It was all getting way beyond the realms of reality, I couldn't confide in anybody but my fear increased and a new wave of terror consumed me. I now felt I was being punished for all the bad things I had done and all the sins I had committed. The chickens had really come home to roost. I started to see the pain in others and blamed myself and somehow linked it to me. I believed the tables had turned and it was now time for me to meet my maker. The feeling of despair faded and was replaced with fear. Just like when the previous drunken nights events hit you one after another my entire life's memory of bad things emptied its contents in my brain. All I could think about was when I had done that, or when I had said that. There was no respite, it was relentless. Although I hadn't done anything majorly bad, I was no angel and had been pretty careless over the years but who hasn't? I couldn't see any rational, in my eyes I soon viewed myself as evil. Soon external events were happening and I linked them back to me, I would take on the responsibility for all the bad in the world and believed it was somehow linked to me. I didn't know why but I had this awful feeling that people had become angry with the world and they wanted change. The problem was I believed the only way to rid the world of this evil was to extract me from existence.

After work had sent me home I went back after a few days, again this just exemplifies how indivisible mental illness really is. One day I took my brother into University, but didn't go into work, I dropped Alex off and then made my way home. Alex at this time was studying Real Estate at Hallam University. I would always look up to my brother, he seemed to have got everything I wanted, he had a number of lovely girlfriends, good career path and a much better way about him, I really wanted to be just like him. On the way into town I wasn't talking but I did say I wanted to be a different person and Alex said

'You can be, everyone can change'.

Unfortunately I was too far gone for such wise words to be absorbed. I dropped him off and then headed back towards Aston. I'd not slept for probably 2 weeks around this point and god only knows how I was capable of driving. If you have a late night you feel tired the next day when driving but no sleep for weeks is another level.

I had made my mind up, today was the day I was going to end my life. The problems in my head were now far beyond a depressed state, I knew help was not an option and that my issues were a consequence of the choices I had made and there was not a single soul on earth who could help me. I knew my fate was in the hands of powers far beyond the restrictions of the world. I had nobody to help me, it was me against everyone and everything and I knew this was a battle where I would not be victorious. I stopped off at a car dealers to see how much they would give me for my Golf. I decided I was going to sell my car before ending my life. I had large debts and I knew by me ending my life would not only cause devastation on a grand scale but everyone else around me would be left to pick up the financial pieces and of course I had no money for a funeral. I had previously visited the NatWest with whom I had the loan with and without putting it bluntly I asked them what would happen if I died. The answer was my parents would not be responsible for the debt. Even if they would have said they were it would not have swayed by decision, I was too far down the line. My student loan would have been written of and the credit cards I expect would have too. I did have a few savings as before I became ill I had managed to lodge a complaint against the Halifax bank who had totally miss sold my Grandma an investment bond, the lovely lady at the Halifax thought it would be ethically and morally just to invest my Grandmothers entire savings into some high risk investment fund. When stocks went South in 2008 she lost 30% or so due to her exposure to UK and International Equities. David constructed me a letter and we sent it to the Halifax, in the end they gave her back the full money she lost plus any interest she lost whilst not having the money in a deposit account. The result was she got back thousands and she kindly gave me a cut. It's strange, I spent every other penny that came into my hands but never spend that money from my Grandma.

It turned out the guy at the dealers didn't want my car and I think he was a bit shocked at how desperate I was to sell it but he never bought it plus of course I didn't have the log book. I made my way to Dels in Swallownest near to where I lived and bought myself a 6 pack of John Smiths, a bottle of vodka, a couple of scratch cards and a pack of Chilli Heatwave Dorito's. I made my way to Aston Ponds which was a fishing place very close to where I grew up and parked my Golf. As kids we used to ride our bikes around there and Richard's parents own the fields surrounding it so I knew it well plus it was the highest bridge I knew of. As soon as I got out of my car my phone rang, I answered it. It was David. I spoke for a short amount of time and he said there are no major problems at work except for the stock market collapsing, I didn't get the joke and believed him and thought it was related to me. He advised me to go for a walk around a golf course. This was good advice but unfortunately I was too far past that. By this point I had come to the conclusion that my whole life was being watched and my every move was being monitored. I thought they knew where I was going and timed the call just to get me when I started walking. I was fully convinced every aspect of my life was now tapped. It then suddenly dawned on me that my whole life since birth had been watched and every bad thing I had ever done had been noted. As each moment passed life became worse and worse and the extent of my problems became universal. I believed all eyes were now on me. I then headed up the hillside and climbed out of the ponds area and made my way to the motorway bridge. It was drizzling and very cloudy, just one of those damp miserable days. I had my work shoes on which had a hole in them, the grass leading to the bridge was very long and soon after I set of my feet and legs became soaked. It took about 20 minutes to get to the bridge, all sorts was going through my head. I was naturally scared about what was going to happen and feared the consequences for everyone I knew. But somehow whilst walking to the bridge I found a little bit of peace amongst the despair. I knew that shortly the suffering would be over. That feeling of peace didn't last very long and I soon was jolted back into reality. I knew that although I might escape my pain of this world I would not be able to do this eternally. Of course the way my brain worked meant that I would always be at the bottom, eventually the thought of suicide filled me with fear as by now I had come to the conclusion that my evil was wicked beyond belief. However I did not have a choice, my decision was final. At the top of the hill there is a farm house and you keep walking over the field then you make your way up a steep embankment and you eventually find yourself on the bridge. It was the bridge over the M1 just near the turn of for junction 31 (Northbound) signposted Worksop, I would jump from the bridge into the North bound traffic. This is where I had decided my existence on this world would cease. I had my Versace jeans on which I used to wear when I was 17, they no longer fitted me but I had lost so much weight that they did now. I also had my Barbour coat on and Burberry T-Shirt. I wanted to be found in my best clothes. I took with me a pen and paper to write a message. Once I was on the bridge I started drinking the cans and having a couple of slurps of the vodka, I was drinking them really fast. As I was scared of jumping I thought the alcohol would give me the confidence to actually step of the edge. At first the vodka was awful to drink neat but it soon became acceptable as I knew I needed it to carry out my final act. I started writing my suicide note and for the first time in years I started to cry. I cried my eyes out. I was thinking about how I was going to miss my family and the realisation that I would never see their faces again, how much I had failed in life and so badly that I wished things could have been different for everyone. I so badly didn't want this to be the end of my life, I had so much to give and so much to offer but I was misunderstood. People didn't know the real me, I was just a burden and I was no use to anybody. I was sad because I think I knew deep down that I had tried and I was sad for myself, it was such a waste of life and such a disastrous end for everyone involved. It wasn't fair on me. I was saying goodbye to every single person I loved, I hadn't even said goodbye or told them how much I cared for them. Instead my true feelings for everyone I cared for and the wider world in general were about to disappear forever. I had given so much to the people around me and I felt I didn't receive the same back. People had often mocked me, called me gay or taken me for a fool but I wasn't. I was just a person trying to find his way in life, there was always somebody who had to work against you. That's life though isn't it? But at the time I couldn't understand it, how come not everyone treats others with the respect they deserve. It's because this world is one messed up place and for a lot of people the only way they feel happiness is at the expense of others. Well that's fine, it's a fact of life but I couldn't cope with that, I wanted things to be different but the world has to be like that for it to work. I just wanted to feel happiness like everyone else in the world. I wanted to be loved and to give love back in return.

I had written a good few pages in my notepad, I went through all my family members and close friends and individually wrote a few lines about them and how they had affected my life in a good way. I had received a lot of love from them over the years but for whatever reason that was not enough. I could not have asked for anything else from them and often wonder how I became in this mess. I think I tried to explain myself but I couldn't really put my feelings into words, especially not in that state. I did however know this note would be the last thing people heard from me and would be the only thing left of me. Within the note I accepted that I had failed in life, I did stress though that I did try. There was no way I could turn things around, I drank all 6 of my cans and had drank a lot of the vodka. I took the scratch cards in the hope that I may win some money to cover funeral costs. Of course I didn't. The rain got heavier and by this point my whole body was drenched. Once the note was finished and my beer had been drank my heart started beating faster and faster as I knew what was going to happen. My final goodbyes had been said, I now realised that these were the last remaining moments of my life and very shortly my body would be an empty vessel and my soul would move onto another realm. I sat there still sobbing with tears rolling down my cheeks one after another the time was upon me. I was about to make my way to the edge. Then across the other side of the bridge I could see a figure walking towards me dressed in Black with a hood up. I sat there, I couldn't move. The figure got closer and closer. She just starred straight at me. As she got close she walked straight past me and continued looking ahead, as if I wasn't there. As she passed me she said

"You're having a nice party aren't you"

And that was it. There were beer cans, a vodka bottle and a note pad strewn across a motorway bridge and that's all she could say. There was nothing else from this woman just those few words. That kind of summarises life, nobody out there can help you only yourself.

This women had knocked me of course, I had lost all my momentum and focus which I had built up for sometime. I walked away from the bridge and made my way to a little wooded section and hid from the police as I was convinced they were going to turn up. I mean what kind of lady sees a young man on a bridge and doesn't phone for help? I remember being stuck in the trees and catching my coat on a thorn and for some strange reason my thinking changed a little. A slight wave of different emotion now came over me, nothing major but given my critical state of mind even the smallest of change in frame of mind made a significant change to my pending fate.

I made my way further away from the bridge and just stood in a trance. I remember thinking I am still alive, I haven't died. Maybe a sense of relief passed through me I'm not sure. After sometime of being in a daze I then turned my phone on. My Mum had been trying to ring me many times, work had phoned her as I hadn't turned up and they were obviously concerned for my welfare. There were several missed calls and messages and in the end I answered her call and she asked me where I was. I told her I was near to my old school, I informed her that I had just been walking. She said she would come right away and pick me up. I stumbled all the way across the fields and back towards home, I went a totally different way home and got lost. I was covered in mud and my cream trousers were now a shade darker, I was very drunk and smelt of liquor. I stashed my bottle of vodka and bag full of empty cans in a gateway just near to where the fields end and the housing estate starts close to my house in Aston. My Mum picked me up in her Corsa and took me home, I cant really remember what I said to her and my head as I'm sure you can imagine was in pieces. I didn't have any emotion, I didn't feel love for anybody anymore, all that was gone. Just a shell remained. I was no longer any use to the world. Tom Gray no longer existed.

24. THE CONSPIRACY

I remember thinking that everything was a set up and the things that were happening in my life were somehow controlled by external factors. For instance on the way up towards the bridge from the ponds where I parked a man asked me what date it was I of course didn't have a clue, I couldn't tell him and to be honest I didn't even know what day it was, I thought he was an actor. I believed the fact that Chad was in prison was a test to see if I would stop him from getting such a long sentence, I thought he wasn't even in prison and it was all staged for me to think he was and all the letters were written by him at home. On my way home after being on the bridge my brother drove past me on a smaller bridge over the A57. How could it be so that he would just by chance pass me whilst I was crossing over the bridge and even notice me and beep? That only happened because something was controlling his actions. At the time I thought he had been instructed by the authorities to drive at that point in time as they knew where I was. I went home after my event on the bridge and tried to sober up. Mum, Alex and Christie were in and they were in the lounge watching X Factor. It was in some foreign country so probably the judge's houses stage and my Mum made me a glass of water and told me to sit with them. So here I was 1 hour after trying my best to hurl myself from a bridge into oncoming traffic, I was back home watching Simon Cowell in his White vest select yet another fantastic Christmas number 1.

Things had now gone from bad to worse. Maybe I had died and this was my eternal punishment.

I'm not sure if my Mum and Dad knew what I had planned to do, to be honest at the time I don't think they did. Eventually my Dad came home and everything was surreal. I remember just not knowing what to do, I just kept drinking glass of water after glass of water. I needed to do something but I didn't know what. My Dad tried talking to me but there were no words left inside me. The function between thought and speech had gone. I no longer thought in a way that people do, my brain was wired. It was deeply infected. As the alcohol wore off the 0.001% better feeling I derived from it evaporated. I then realised that my only method of ending the overpowering fear, suicide, was no longer an option to me. Again my words do not some close to explain the feeling I had within me. There are no words known to us. All the normal describing words do not come close in giving the reader some feeling as to what it felt like to be me at that time, I often never talk about it because when I'm talking I think, no Tom it was much worse than that. There are many people out there who have been to these horrific places within their brains and I'm sure those people may kind of understand.

My Dad went and collected my car from the Ponds where it had been abandoned that afternoon. By this point they were now extremely worried. I still remained untreated and my condition became much worse, it's hard to say why but the power behind my fears grew as each day went by. There was no respite, my brain never stopped spinning. Every second the bombardment of extreme thought was sending electricity into my brain. My eyes grew wider and eventually my mind and body became possessed. Something had now taken over, my shell had now become a vehicle that was transporting another force. This feeling of such negative energy within me grew and grew. The energy that now engulfed me was dark and twisted. I was convinced that I was going to get punished for the things I at the time deemed to be 'bad' because after all what we do in life echoes in eternity. This wasn't just a minor punishment but a global force that was not only going to punish me for the things I had done but were also going to frame me for crimes I had not committed. As the forces I was fighting were so great I had no power in stopping them. For instance I took my car in to get repaired so that the electric window could get sorted, I was convinced my parents had asked the mechanic to stash drugs in the inside of the car. I was convinced they were trying to frame me so that I would end up in prison. In addition to that my Grandma had given me some fertilizer for the grass and I also thought they were trying to make out I was making bombs with it.

I thought I was a very bad person and as I looked back on my life and all I could see was the negative side, I couldn't see any of the good things that I had done. My Mum was trying to make me feel better about myself and asked me "what are your good qualities?" and I couldn't think of any. My reply was "cutting grass" then even after I said that I managed to talk myself around so that I wasn't even good at that. I could see not one good part to me. For some reason even after the events on the bridge I was still driving and went into work despite my condition was getting far worse. I didn't last and went home, my parents realised it wasn't helping me. My parents weren't sure what was the matter with me, it's hard to imagine that nobody could see any of this, my mind had gone and in its place was something else. I don't know how things could get any worse, I'm sure other people go through worse things but for me looking back my life had become the root of all evil in the world. I believed I was evil and I knew that every person in the world knew all along and that they had all been nice to me all these years waiting for the time when I would be punished. The time for such punishment was now upon me. I had been set up well and truly and thought I had been chosen to be the carrier of such badness in the world. I knew everyone wanted me banishing, when people would talk to me but I knew deep down they hated every part of me. It's a strange place to be, right at the bottom. I believed that all the horrendous people in the world were somehow better than me and that there crimes were somehow part of a much greater plot.

I somehow believed that all the evil in the world was not real but instead a cover up to pull me in. I had been well and truly caught and I had taken the bate at every opportunity. Unbelievable that it is I was still driving at this point and gave my parents a lift to a Halloween party. The party was at the Yellow Lion and before going out my Dad jokingly said here put this mask on, it was a pride of chucky mask along with a plastic knife. I obviously didn't want too but had no fight left in me so put it on. Of course everyone laughed when I put it on, the fear I had inside me was immense. I took them up to the pub which is only a 5 minute drive from my house, the pub looked rammed and there was even a coach dropping people off. I pulled in the car park and stopped as far away from the door as I could. My honest belief was everyone in the pub was there for me, they would be getting drunk all talking about what they were going to do to me. I believed I was going to be taken from my house and taken to a big disused warehouse where everything was set up. I would be bundled into this place with a bag over my head, I would then be tied down to a chair. Then the bag would be removed and all the instruments would be exposed. There was going to be a big screen where I would be shown the highlights of my life, as my whole life had been watched from birth all my sins would be shown for the world to see. My Nannan had been poorly around this time but I wasn't informed for obvious reasons. The night before this my Dad came through the room with a box of something, I asked him what it was and he just said something like its just some pork pie. I believed this was going to be my last supper, they were going to ram pork pie down my throat as a way of saying how much of a greedy pig I was. After I had watched the video I would then be subject to long and enduring torture techniques from all the people I had offended over the years. I wanted to run, there was nowhere to hide. I wanted to speak to somebody, there was nobody. This was it. I had an entire population hungry for my death. They didn't want me to die quickly, they wanted a slow and painful death..

On they way to the pub my Mum said that I should go see my Grandma who lives a few roads away from us, I thought my Mum wanted me to see my Grandma before I was taken away, maybe so she could tell me something. I called in after dropping off Chucky and Co. She made me a drink and had lit loads of candles, this might have been to create a tranquil environment, either that or she hadn't paid her bill again. I sat and drank tea, she offered me her spare bed and wanted me to stop. I felt safe there, she said she would make me a hot chocolate and I could try and get some sleep. I so wanted to stop however I knew tomorrow would come. I wanted it over with. For the last few weeks I just kept saying, give me one more day with my family. By now I wanted to walk that Green Mile and face the music.

I stepped out of my Grandmas house for what felt like the last time, I knew I would never see her again. I said something to her as I was leaving like 'I cant hide forever', I then turned and headed into the night. I went back to my empty house, got in bed and waited. I didn't turn the light of, I kept hearing noises outside, I knew somebody was there. I lay on my bed for hours, it wasn't if they were coming it was when. Time went slowly and of course nobody came. My Mum and Dad returned. Naturally they thought it would be a good idea to come into my room with their costumes on. Christie also came home around this time and she had done something to her tongue and said it felt like it had been chopped of, I believed she was talking in code and this was something else that was going to happen to me. Everyone went to bed, I just lie there. Waiting. I would hate it when the sun rose, I knew another day of torment lay ahead.

Richard by this point was ringing me everyday. He'd asked hopefully 'are you feeling any better today?' Of course I wasn't. Some days I'd say yeah a little just to show some willing but inside I was slowly drifting further. It's hard to imagine how things could get any worse. But they did. They say that what doesn't kill you makes you stronger. The fact is it had killed me.
Richard would often take me out in his van, he'd ask if I wanted to go out and I of course didn't because of the very fact I believed everyone wanted me hung drawn and quartered. But I'd say, yeah I'll come out because I knew hiding was no longer an option. One time he took me down to a gypsy camp to make a delivery and I was convinced they were going to lock me in a stable and tie me up, they would then chop my arms of one by one until I confessed

to what I had done. I thought people had said things about gypsies whilst I was there and recorded it. Because I didn't step in and stand up for the gypsies I believed they thought I had disrespected them. For this reason they wanted to punish me. This wasn't just gypsies but every community from disabled people to different ethnic groups, etc. There was nobody on earth who I hadn't upset. The problem I had was I hadn't really done anything wrong, I remember thinking they're going to torture me forever as I wouldn't have anything to confess too. I live next to a large playing fields and they were digging a load of soil out so that water could be stored there instead of running straight into the stream at the bottom of the field to prevent flooding further down stream. I thought they were building an English equivalent of I'm A Celebrity Get Me Out Of Here and I was going to be the one who was starring in it. I thought they were going to do tasks where they tortured me and after they had tortured me they were going to bury me alive. Along the trenches there were loads of T shapes. I of course thought that was to show me where I was going. I think these T shapes are used for surveying purposes.

I was convinced I was a bad person so I was doing things to try and stop getting tortured and make me a better person, one thing I would do was pick up rubbish whenever I was out, this was in some way to make myself a better person, so I'd go out with the dog for example and come back with a handful of rubbish. This one time I went out and picked up about 10 pieces of dog excrement and put it all in the dog bin. I was convinced everything was a test, for example my Grandma asked me to fill her washers up in her car, I had to get everything right so I got a measuring jug and did it all to the exact measurements I also was convinced that my grandma had done something to her car and that I had to find out what was wrong with it. If I didn't I thought the car was going to crash when she went on the motorway, so I was looking all around her car looking for items that were wrong. I don't have a clue about cars so failed that little test. When my mum and dad were working my Grandma would come over to look after me, I was paranoid and was convinced something bad was going to happen. We were changing bulbs in the kitchen and I thought someone had set it up so when I touched the bulb I would get an electric shock. Another time my Mum asked me to feed the cat, right next to the food was a sharp fork like instrument that I had never seen before. It was just sticking up and it nearly caught my hand. Before things got really bad I snapped one of my golf clubs in anger, so my Dad thought it would be a good idea to get it mended for me so we took it to the local driving range where they fixed clubs. As I wasn't thinking straight I was convinced they were going to put my hand in the vice and chop my fingers of, this was for messing about in the driving range when I was younger. You can see how my whole world became one of survival, I'd survive having my fingers chopped off but something else would take its place. I was frantically trying to find out who I was, I wanted there to be at least some purpose to my life before it ended. I googled my name and it came up with a gay poet from the 18th Century which of course fuelled the theory that I believed everyone thought I was gay.

I wanted to find something to cling on too so when the physical pain commenced I could think of that but there was nothing. This would make the pain far greater. I would look at pictures from when I was a child and see things that weren't there, I would look at people in the photos and think they were taking the piss out of me behind my back. My Grandma did a tapestry made out of cross stitch for us and it hangs on our stairs. On it it details all our three names (The Gray Siblings) with dates of birth and times of birth. She also stitched 2 flowers next to each of our names but she only did 1 next to my name. I believed there was an ulterior motive behind this subtle difference and that it was because she knew I was bad. I thought my Mum had been chosen to raise the devil as they knew how strong a person she is. Then once I was destroyed she would receive her reward for taking on this burden.

When I was working at Westcourt one of the clients phoned up and said something and referred to me as Dorian Grey and he said

"That's a bit of general knowledge for if you are in a quiz".

"It is about a handsome man and that I too was handsome".

Now that stuck in my mind for some reason and when I became ill towards the end of October I googled the film and looked what it was about and it was about a young man who loses his looks as this painting slowly gets ruined. So I thought that he was indicating that this would happen to me. Strangely enough I had a caricature of myself in my bedroom, this wasn't on my wall but leant on my wall on the floor. The next thing the picture of me becomes damaged and the frame is broken so I thought this is what will happen to me. Mum in her wisdom went to get a new frame for the picture but it was smaller than the original one and so my legs had to be chopped of as they wouldn't fit in the new frame. I couldn't believe this and was petrified. I was 100% sure that now my legs at some point would removed. My Mum of course told me I was being stupid but to me it was my truth, what are the chances of a man saying such a random film to me when were weren't even talking about anything relating to that and then my picture gets damaged. Another time my Grandma asked me to stake one of her trees in her garden, I was hammering it in and every time I struck the wood I told myself this is what will happen to me. I could feel the pain within me with every blow.

These distorted ideas went on for a good few weeks, on bonfire night my local pub, The Yellow Lion were having a bonfire and fireworks, I was invited and a few friends told me to go up, in my deluded state I was convinced that I was going to be a real life Guy Fawkes and that I was going to get burned alive, I passed on that night believe it or not. I had given up the idea of suicide as I convinced that I was heading straight to hell for my sins that I had committed. My behaviour continued like this and my Mum, Dad and Grandma were unsure what to do until one day in November 2010 when my behaviour reached crisis point. My grandma was round at our house as we were having discussions, they were saying you need to do something. But what could I do? What on earth could somebody in my situation have done? This wasn't a fixable solution. The demise of me was what the world had been waiting for for thousands of years. The point had come in history where the people could become free and end all of the misery. It was just unfortunate that that person would have to be me. My dad came home to drop the car off before he went for a quick drink at the pub. I was pacing around the room and when my dad got home I said to them

"This is it they've come for me, I'm finished"

I can't put in words how frightened I was, every car that pulled up I believed was the one that was going to take me away forever. Vans were just coming down our road and stopping outside our house, this never happens. My mum decided enough was enough and called for the emergency doctor. He turned up about an hour later. The doctor who came to the house was German and couldn't speak very good English. It felt unreal and that my life was turning out to be something out of a very strange and twisted film. I remember him having to look in this book when it came to what he was prescribing me which was 10mg of Diazepam. By this point I had given up and was just waiting to be taken away, I was literally pulling my hair out with fear and I mean literally, anyway, after the doctor turned up and prescribed some medication I eventually took the pill after a large amount of persuading, I knew once I swallowed the tablet it would be over. I thought that the pill was going to send me to sleep by which time I would be taken away whilst I was asleep and taken to a place to be tortured and pay the eternal price. I took the pill. My Mum asked me to sit down on the sofa and I did. I'm not sure if I fell asleep but a massive rush came over me. It was incredible and intense. Suddenly I had gone back to the real Tom, every single thing I thought had totally vanished from my mind. I was sat down talking to all 3 of them and I was laughing at some of the things I was thinking. I thought gosh that was crazy, I'm so glad its over. All I wanted to do was go out for tea with them all and Richard to thank them for how much they had helped me over the last few months. Richard had been an amazing support, I think a few of my mates didn't know what to say to me, but he did. He even went as far as to see a specialist so that he could help me. At the time it didn't feel like his calls or visits helped as I wanted to be alone. But I think deep down they nestled in my broken heart somewhere and made a subtle, subconscious effect. I told my Dad that I thought I was going to be punished and he said I hadn't done any bad stuff and that he had done bad things too. You know like sell a piece of fillet steak when in fact it was a piece of rump. I made that bit up he didn't say that. But he kind of said we all make mistakes and that I wasn't going to get punished. My Mum then gave the standard Father Son emotion command and said 'give him a hug'. Nobody could believe the change in me in such a short space of time and if my family hadn't been there to witness it then nobody would have believed it. I told them all I was thinking awful things and that I was going to be cut up into pieces and put in a suitcase and sent to Australia. My problems had literally been taken away and I thought I was fixed. Now if people are unsure if mental health problems really exist then how can the addition of some chemical in my brain remove all the pain? That is a strong argument for the chemical in balance theory. It is true yes, talking therapies are more effective than medication for mild depression and I totally agree with that. Feeding the population pills is no answer but unfortunately that is what is happening. GP's just give the stuff out like nobodies business but they are not to blame. There is no education or alternatives. If we all lived in a perfect world we would get specialist treatment and a whole host of therapies but let's get real this isn't going to happen. There is no answer I'm afraid, I wish I had one. The money being generated from the pharmaceutical companies is incredible and a wise woman once told me that money makes the world go round. Pills equal profits, profits equals research, research equals better pills, better pills equals better people, better people equals greater profits. Its like everything in nature, its just a cycle. The problem is you've just got to find out whereabouts you sit.

I've since seen the film Limitless with Bradley Cooper which is about a guy who takes 1 pill and becomes a great success and all his problems disappear, that's what it felt like, I was back to my old self, after being immersed into some other world for months I was suddenly back to the happy person I so badly wanted to be all my life. I told my Grandma I was fine and she said that's great but I should try and go on one of those Dale Carnegies courses (I'd read his books). I said that was a good idea and headed to bed. I couldn't wait to get in bed and sleep as it so long since my eyes had shut and I had rested my battered body. Unfortunately that good feeling only lasted a short time more then as swiftly as it rushed through me it vanished. It happened so quickly, it was like somebody somewhere had switched the switch. The dread and fear soon replaced those distant good feelings. I was back to what felt like hell, or the waiting room just outside hell where I was waiting to enter. I went to bed that night in my clothes, I remember thinking I want to be taken away in some clothes not just in my boxer shorts. I selected Black clothes as I didn't want to see the blood on my clothes when I was tortured. So I went to bed but I still didn't sleep, I was now fully back in the living nightmare which had become my life. By this point I started hallucinating, I could smell things that weren't there. I could smell a strange kind of gas or a burning type of smell.

As time passed it just came on at certain times in the house. I tried telling my parents that there was a strange smell but of course they couldn't smell anything. I thought the whole house had been rigged up and all the smells were being set by some investigators, what they were doing was testing that I cared about my family. So what I thought they were doing was setting the smell off and then monitoring my response. I thought I had to get my family out of the house and get the house checked in order to pass the test. I remember watching a film with my Mum, Brother and Sister and these smells kept coming and going, I remember not doing anything and keeping quiet. I thought that the shower was also faulty and that whoever went in would get electrocuted. For instance I'd have like a 30 second shower as I was so frightened of being electrocuted, at one stage I was banging on the bathroom door telling My Mum to get out of the shower as it was dangerous. The smells didn't go away, the smells of burning kept coming back when I was trying to go to sleep. By this point I was sleeping downstairs or trying to get some sleep at least but was unsuccessful. These smells where coming and going to the point where I went off alarming. Also this night I told my Mum to move as I believed somebody was going to chuck a brick through the window, these were all my thoughts that I thought were reality. It's like something was inside my head saying that someone is outside right now and if you don't move your Mum then she's going to get hit by it. The smells got stronger and more intense, I didn't know what to do. I didn't want to cause a scene but I didn't want anything bad to happen to my family. My head was literally exploding, I had two options and neither was good. I was going insane. I stood up in our longue and faced up to my Dad, I told my him he had to get my sister out of the house, she was sleeping upstairs, I don't think my brother was in that night. So I was shouting and screaming at my Dad saying we are all in danger and if we don't get out we were all going to die. My Mum took me upstairs to show me that my sister was ok but that wasn't good enough. I demanded that we should turn the gas of at which point my Dad got angry and said this all had to stop, I was stood square in his face while I was going off on one. I remember my mum saying your dads a lot bigger than you so I suggest you step down but I couldn't stop myself and my dad had to physically hold me in the lounge to stop me trying to get out of the house into the porch to turn off the gas. I was getting urges that I needed to fight my Dad to prove that I cared and that if I did nothing it showed I was a cowered. I couldn't hit my Dad though and also couldn't leave my sister, the whole situation was putting deep cuts in my mind. The problem was the smells were so real to me but no one else could smell anything. I stepped down after trying to pass the test and accepted defeat knowing my lack of results would lead to further punishment. I was beginning to give up with the tests as I never seemed to pass any, if I did pass one then there was another put right in my tracks. The next day I was at home with my Dad, we were both sat in the living room not doing much. I remember there were so many adverts on TV for charities and they were really graphic, I thought they were being put on my screen to show me how much suffering there is in the world and that I've had it easy and put nothing back in. My Dad even commented about the frequency of these adverts and I thought he was saying something to kind of say look what there putting on telly for you to see. All of a sudden I looked at my Dad and noticed he had fallen asleep so I decided to go into the kitchen and it just so happened that there was a British Gas bill just sat there in the kitchen, I remember thinking this had been planted there so when I walked in the kitchen I'd see it. Anyway I saw it and picked it up and decided to ring the number where it says about smelling gas. My Dad woke up just as I was finishing the call and he couldn't believe what I had done, by this point he was near the end of his tether. He rang the gas board back and said there wasn't a gas leak but by this time it was too late, once an issue has been raised they have to check it out. We both sat there in silence for about 10 minutes then a man turned up from British Gas to try and find a Gas leak that had been created in my head. So he checked the boiler and came with an instrument, what he brought was a long lead with a box at the end and it looked like it plugged into the electric, what I saw however was a piece of torturing equipment, I thought the man and my Dad were going to tie me to a chair and send electric shocks through my body. I wasn't 100% sure what they thought I was going to tell them but I was sure something was going to happen.

While I was unwell I lost total respect for myself which is common with people with severe depression, I would have to be told to wash, shower and look after myself. In this time period my hair grew quite long. So my Dad suggested that I should go to the barbers. As I was extremely paranoid I believed they were going to cut my flesh with their razor. So I sat down in the chair petrified the whole time, especially when they went around my ears. I was just waiting for them to tie me down and start cutting me up. I made a hastily exit. The constant bombardment of danger was continuous however there was one strange lapse of such fear. This was going to the toilet. That was the only time the pain stopped, this may be why they call it relief.

Our new TV went a bit funny, a red mark appeared on the left side of the screen and before long it disappeared. So my Mum rang the place where we got the TV and an engineer came out. What he did was lay the TV on its back and start taking parts out one by one, he also gave us a running commentary. What I saw was what was going to happen to me, I believed they were going to take my organs out one by one just like the man was doing taking parts out of the TV. My mum said to the man "it seems to get worse when the judges are on X Factor" why on earth she came up with that conclusion I'll never know. Maybe she studied Electronics at University and never told me. So from that I thought it was a sign that I was being judged and the red indicated bad.

By this point I had convinced myself I was the extreme of bad, I was in fact a human equivalent of the devil. Things just spiralled out of control and my thoughts were getting very farfetched. I came up with the theory that here on earth is a test for the actual real world and what happens here is an assessment. I believed that in the real world there is no suffering and this is just a filter system. Everything that happens to you is arranged and there are no coincidences.

It's funny how coincidence plays a big part in people's lives in general, things happen and we try to find patterns and link things together. I thought that my whole life had been mapped out for me and there was no way I could change things. For instance a few days after I had tried to turn the gas of because I could smell it I was sat in our longue watching the news with my Mum and Grandma. The top story was there was a gas leak in Manchester and it had blown up some houses and caused a major problem. Luckily nobody had died on this occasion. Now what a coincidence that was. All I can smell is gas then there is a serious explosion. What I saw was *you could have prevented this*. It was around this time that I thought the television was about me and all the newspaper headlines were linked to me. For instance I could flick through a whole paper and instantly think of a time when I had done something related to a given headline. No thinking time the link just appeared in my brain. I remember watching Loose Women at home and Russell Brand was on, I thought they were all laughing and joking about me and making fun out of me. I remember on the show thinking that at any point I would become live on the show and that all the hidden cameras would be shown to the general public.

I thought that everything that was bad in the world was my fault, I blamed myself for the recession we were in, blamed myself for my Dad's shop been quiet, I thought once they had got rid of me the world would become a better place; for example I thought the world economy would vastly improve and that all things would go back to how they were in the so called 'good times'. For instance they would get rid of speed cameras and that everyone would stop committing crime. I even thought at one point that people's relatives who had died would come back to life as they had not actually died but had gone somewhere until I had gone. I'm sure this is difficult to understand but it was all completely 'real' to me and shows how poorly a persons mind can become.

A couple of days after the German doctor had been round I had a meeting with my own GP, which wasn't my usual doctor. I went in the doctors and it felt everyone's eyes were on me, as I thought it was all staged I thought the people who were at the docs were people I had offended in the past. There was this one bloke who is a driving instructor and I once threw a snowball at his car, anyway he got out and pinned me up against some conifers and said it could have had a rock in it. Well he was there, staring at me. The doc was ginger, and as I've sometimes joked about the ginger community I thought it was another sign to say we know you have disrespected the ginger army. She agreed I was suffering from some sort of depression and referred me to a specialist in the Mental Health Department (this referral letter finally arrived with an appointment at home in January 2011 – 2 months after my episode). Who knows what would have happened to me if I was left untreated until then.

My Mum and Dad knew something was very wrong and that I needed immediate help but didn't know what to do. If it was a physical illness people would have been able to see how much I was hurting. Unbeknown to me they had been speaking with people in the mental health field for weeks before. I kept very quiet so all the things I was thinking I kept to myself and on the surface I just seemed very down. My Mum knew a lady who worked in Mental Health and in desperation she phoned her up and asked her what to do and she was told to tell the doctors that she feared for my life and insist that the Crisis Team were involved. My GP came out to our house later that afternoon and said that there was obviously a problem and that he would refer me immediately to the Crisis Team. Two men came out to our house within the hour and after a couple of hours talking to me they were convinced I was having a psychotic episode, my diagnosis around this point was Psychotic Depression. The Crisis Team are a group of people who operate when people are in a time of need, a time of crisis with regards their mental health. I didn't know who these people were and was extremely paranoid. I thought they were from the church and that eventually they were going to take me somewhere. As I thought they could read my mind I couldn't even hide my own thoughts, I had no privacy my entire life and mind had totally been taken away from me. As something was inside my mind they knew exactly what I didn't like and what would cause me the most discomfort. This way when the punishment commenced they could target the areas of most pain with pin point accuracy. I told them everything about my life and told them all the things I wouldn't want anyone to know. I thought if I just tell the whole truth then I won't be lying to them and make matters worse. The Team wanted to hospitalise me but my Mum and Dad said they were happy to look after me at home and that I had a 24 hour watch on me by my parents. They took it in turns to sleep in my room by the door so that if I got up it would wake them up. I was started on some medication, they started me on 10mg Citalopram and 10mg Olanzapine and we were told that it would take 3 weeks for the medication to kick in, the medication didn't work at first so they increased my Citalopram from 10mg to 20mg and the Crisis Team called daily to the house to check how I was reacting to the drugs.

The Citalopram adds Serotonin into your brain, Serotonin is a chemical that relays signals between brain cells. During such episodes a person's brain can produce higher levels of Dopamine. Dopamine is also a chemical within the brain and Olanzapine alters the levels of it within your brain. To keep things simple and also because I don't fully understand it lets just say the 2 drugs adjust the chemicals in my brain to a more stable level. Olanzapine is also used to treat people with Schizophrenia and I can't really see where the line is drawn between a psychotic episode and Schizophrenia. However I am sure there are some major medical differences I am unaware of.

Eventually I slept a little as the Olanzapine also acts as a sedative. In total I didn't sleep for 3 weeks and I mean not even a wink. Sleep depravation is used as a torture technique and that is what I was doing to myself. People don't believe me when I tell them how long I didn't sleep for but it is the truth.

I was purely surviving on adrenaline, my eyes never shut for the whole time, I tell a lie, I remember once in the car my eyes shut for about 3 seconds and that was the sum total of my rest. I must have lost around two stone in weight around autumn 2010.

The Olanzapine was made by a pharmaceutical company called Lilly and it said this on the white tablet along with a number underneath. I believed it was referring to Lilly Allen who had been having a bad time in the papers etc and I thought I was responsible. I read all the side effects of the medication and I believed that I would get all of them and this was my punishment. In addition to this Cheryl Cole was in the news for nearly dying from Malaria and as I didn't have any injections when I went to Thailand it was god's way of showing me what my carelessness has caused. (For the record I had blood tests for everything upon my return to the UK and was all clear plus was I extremely careful against other infections).

It was now well into November and the winter was a very bad one. I remember one time my Mum and Grandma taking me for a walk around Clumber Park, I was still very poorly at this stage and very paranoid. Again coincidences come into play here, for some reason the roads were very busy, I had never noticed the roads being so busy before mid-week. I thought they were all coming to Clumber Park to witness me being publically executed. When we got to Clumber Park we got out of the car and we headed towards the lake where we started to walk around, just as we started walking around the lake a women came out of the trees screaming her child's name saying she had lost her, now I thought this was a test and that I had to find the missing child, however I then thought if I went to look for the child I was a paedophile. By this point amongst all the other evil things in the world I had also convinced myself I was a paedophile which I am told is not uncommon with people going through an episode. The intrusive thoughts in my head were telling me I was. If I was having these awful thoughts then surely I was this bad person and it was in fact real. After all they were my thoughts and they were created within my head. So I was in a very tricky situation, one where whatever I did was wrong, so I did nothing. If I went looking for the child then I thought people would believe I was in fact a paedophile. If I did nothing then the people would think I didn't care about missing children. Again this sent me crazy as there was no right choice for me to make, every decision I made was the wrong one. Fortunately the child was found pretty quickly. We then drove to a place called The Dukeries, this is an old stately home with an art gallery and a café. In the grounds is a big open fire pit, for want of a better description. I was adamant that I was going to be strapped to the metal objects in the middle of this pit, gas would fill the metal pipes which my arms and legs were wrapped around, they would then ignite the gas and burn my body to death. I think the fear element had left me now, I just wanted the pain to commence. I knew there was nothing on earth I could do to buy me any eternal sanctuary. I began to feel like everyone was just teasing me now and it would take years until I finally get tortured. This was because they could see in my mind and they knew I wanted it over with.

I was so unwell at this stage that I thought my own parents were trying to poison me, I thought they were controlling my actions by putting certain chemicals in my food and in my drinks. It was so bad that when my Mum bought me some vitamins because I had become so frail, I was convinced that they had heroin in them, but of course they were just normal vitamins. I refused to take them and tried flushing them down the toilet, my Mum was very upset to find out that I thought she was poisoning me – this was the last straw for her. I thought she wanted to get me addicted to these drugs and then they would take them away from me and lock me in my room like on Trainspotting. The Crisis Team came to see me every day for most of November but it was a very frightening time for me and for all my close family. On this one occasion my Uncle Mark came over to look after me as my Mum was going back to work and he decided to do some cooking and we went to Sainsburys at Crystal Peaks. I was still really paranoid thinking that everyone was looking at me, I even remember my Uncle asking me whether or not we should buy some Charlotte potatoes and I thought he was hinting that I would like them as they are a girls name and as I was convinced I was a paedophile I thought he was trying to say something. It turned out it was national sausage week and I thought this too was about me, I believed they were going to cut my penis of and cook it in a casserole. I'd never heard of national sausage week and I haven't heard of it since either. In the recipe he used it says in the book you need to hit the meat with a frying pan, so I did this and I could feel that this is what people were going to do with me. On a separate occasion my uncle took me out into the Peak District to get some logs and we managed to get the van stuck, I thought he was testing me to see if I cared about him and his belongings, I thought he wanted me to say no the terrain is too tricky and we should turn back. As it happened luckily enough a tractor was passing and it pulled us out. I of course thought this was all a set up and everyone was in on it. My Uncle also took me to the Yorkshire Sculpture Park and I was extremely paranoid, I thought he was taking me to see exhibits and that they were all aimed at me. For example this one piece of work was called the Gates of Hell and was a massive wooden sculpture plus there were other important pieces of art work which had important meanings too me. I obviously believed it was meant for me to see as I was going to hell. All the way around I was waiting to be captured and taken away, I was so frightened it was untrue but I never showed it. Mark and I walked around the grounds and we were talking and I kept saying I'm a really bad person and that I've done lots of bad things. My Uncle replied with *"so have I, I've also done things I regret"* but that wasn't good enough for me as I was too convinced that I was too bad for this world and I was going to get punished. At one stage I believed I was going to get put on a rocket and projected into outer space and never return. This was because my Dads friend Mick months earlier jokingly said why don't we send Tom into space in a cardboard box, just any 'off the cuff' remarks would send my thoughts racing.

Richard picked me up one time to go out on a delivery with him and my Mum thought it would be a good idea for me to get out of the house, earlier that day my Mum said to me *"What have you done that's so bad?* (As all I kept saying was I'm a really bad person) *"What would you tell me if I was going to saw your arm off?"* Anyway I had no answer to the question as I hadn't done anything bad, so I went out and got in the van and what was there on the floor but a rusty old saw. What are the chances of that? So I believed I was going to be taken away and that the saw was going to be used to saw my arm off. Richard's Dad Sammy who is a great guy *said "why don't you come over for tea and we can have a chat"*. I declined the offer as I believed he, like everybody else, was against me. I remember thinking I would love so much to go round to their house and speak to him and make everything all right but there wasn't anything to fix. I was broken beyond repair. I was so alone in this time period, there was nobody I trusted, nobody I could turn too, and it was me against the whole world.   Plus of course I was fighting forces far beyond the boundaries of this world.

25. CALMER SEAS AHEAD?

As time progressed and I didn't get tortured or captured I began to feel a little, and I mean a little, bit more confident in going out, plus the medication started to work. Now there is some debate as to what made me feel better, was it that the natural cycle of my depression had passed and that I was feeling a bit better? Or was it the medication or even something else? There is only one answer to that one really in my opinion. My psychologist thinks it's more down to thought processes and my psychiatrist thinks it's more down to the medication. My own personal opinion is that it was more down to the medication because I was so ill that nobody could tell me anything, I could have seen the best professionals in the world but at my worst I was convinced I was the devil. Now I don't think any psychologist could have talked me down from that. That was my truth. I have since spoke with a few people about my recovery and people think it was solely down to the meds and I'd probably agree.

After the day at Clumber Park the medication seemed to slowly start to work, I was still having the fear of being taken away but it was much more mellow, the thoughts didn't just disappear they were just a lot quieter. I didn't really change my thinking patterns or do much in regards of making myself better, I did read an Anthony Robbins book called Awaken the Giant that my mother wanted me to read but I don't think the reading played any part in my recovery. December came and things started to improve a little more but I still had very little energy and all I wanted to do was lay in bed for as long as possible. I can remember before getting really unwell I would wake up really early in the mornings, then the next week even earlier. My sleep pattern just deteriorated from there. All I wanted to do was eat and lie in bed, they say that you lose your appetite when you are poorly but I certainly didn't. Once the Olanzapine kicked in my appetite went through the roof, I was craving carbohydrates and sweet stuff, I've got a sweet tooth anyway but this was something else. I just couldn't get enough of food. Apart from the eating I pretty much fitted the criteria for being depressed, I felt hopeless, felt guilty for things I had done in my past, I lacked motivation, I struggled making decisions and I was getting very little enjoyment out of life, so I fitted the bill quite well. At the time I was convinced that something awful was going to happen. The problem was I had no one to run to, I thought my own family was poisoning me and I trusted no one. At my worst I thought people could read my mind, again back to coincidences, somebody would say something and I developed a very efficient and quick way of bringing whatever they said back to me. For example someone would say "she's got a big nose" and I would then think, I was thinking that and they've only just said that to show me they are reading my mind. I continued with the visits and was introduced to the Early Intervention Team once the Crisis Team were happy with my progress. I continued to progress through December. I was not well by any means but a little bit better than I had been, we went to the local pub for a few drinks for my Dads 50th at the end of November. I had a few pints of bitter that night and kept myself away from everyone as I wanted to avoid conversation, I was still very paranoid but a little bit less than I had been. At the time I didn't think I was getting any better but looking back I slowly was getting my health back. There was a lot of snow that winter and all the roads were blocked, Richard even used to go out in his tractor to free up peoples roads. My Dad rang Richard up and he came to our road. He decided it would be a good idea to drive down someone's drive to clear the snow, it was a steep drive. So he went down it but couldn't get out and his wheels were just spinning. I thought it was a test to see if I cared about his machinery so I was frantically digging snow from behind him to try and free his wheels up. He was spinning all over and the bucket on the tractor nearly knocked the roof of this couples porch. He eventually got out. When I was still really poorly my Dad thought it would be a good idea for me to go and help the landlady and landlord out at the pub who as a family we all knew fairly well. So they put me in the function room upstairs on my own and got me painting all of their walls. Around this time I was still expecting my imminent death and didn't exactly try with the edging in. I even painted the wooden bits and there was varnish everywhere, I'm not a good painter at the best of times. They even put some music on and it was all this religious stuff and I thought they wanted me to hear the words in the song which of course I listened too intently. They offered me drinks and some lunch but I believed they were poisoning me and declined their offer. They then asked me to go down the cellar and sweep up, I knew why they wanted me to go down, it was so they could lock me up down there. So I climbed the ladder and went in the cellar and did some sweeping, it was the fastest sweeping session ever conducted. The snow was so bad this day nobody could get to work so everyone went to the pub. I was hiding in the function room upstairs as I didn't want anybody to see me. Then all these kids ran up and were talking to me, then there Mums came up and told their children to go back downstairs. Eventually I had to walk through the pub covered in paint, the pub was so busy, it had never been as busy. As the staff couldn't get to work the customers were serving themselves. I had to get out, all of these people were tipping me over the edge and I felt very anxious. When I walked through the bar it felt like they were all starring at me. I saw Aidan my old school friend but I didn't have anything to say to him I just said hello and left. It was awful. I also thought they were filming me working so they could send the footage to the police for benefit fraud. Whilst I was unwell I did not receive any sick pay from Westcourt just the Statutory Sick Pay of £80 from the state. This crippled my finances further.

It was around this time that I received a call from Chad who gave me some invaluable advice. Prior to this I had very little contact with my friends as I didn't want to talk to them but when my phone rang I answered on this occasion. Through his own experiences he told me without knowing my own circumstances what was going on in my head. He said you will probably thinking........and probably thinking that.........and everything he said was correct. He told me that it will pass and not to worry. To hear those words meant a lot to me especially at a time when I felt nobody knew how I was feeling. I owe Chad a lot for that brief phone call we had whilst I was walking down The Chase to our house. I can remember it like it was yesterday.

My improvement in health got better, it took a while. Before I was better I went back to work, I was still pretty bad but I went anyway. I was very paranoid. I walked down to the bus with an employee called Dave and he was telling me about his daughter who had mental health problems and he specified what it was she suffered with. It turned out it was exactly the same as what I had been diagnosed with and the medication was the same however I thought he was trying to show me that he was in on the act and that he knew everything about me and what was going on in my head.

I continued to go to work on reduced hours and slowly the dark clouds lifted a little, the storm hadn't past but the thick dark grey cumulonimbus clouds had. I remember ringing my old friend Sam up and chatting, I was convinced he was going to be part of all the torture for not helping him enough with his own life. It was such a relief to ask him *'do you want to hurt me'* and him reply *'no'*. I remember getting well on 22nd December, that's when it finally clicked that no one was going to take me away and all the problems that I had created in my mind were not true. I remember this night well. I was at home with Danny and a few other friends watching The Beach and having a few beers. It was like a revelation, the final clouds suddenly lifted from my world and I could see Blue sky for the first time in a long while. I seem to view my recovery like it happened in an instant but when I talk to my family they inform me I got well over the course of a few weeks but either way the recovery time was very quick. It was probably 10 weeks from the day on the bridge back in October. The care I received was fantastic but more importantly the medication I now had within me was essential. I had 6 weeks off work in total and went back full time in January 2011 after a phased return to work over the end of December and after Christmas.

My mood went from being very low and suicidal to 10 weeks later I was as high as a kite. I think it was just sheer relief that I had got my life back after previously convincing myself it was over. It felt like I had taken Ecstasy but good clean stuff and it lasted about 3 weeks. My mood was just through the roof, I remember going to sleep happy and waking up happy too, it never went away. I was just full of life, my energy levels were very high and overall I just felt extremely happy. Its like when you have nightmare and you wake up and realise it wasn't real, but this time the nightmare was in an extreme form and therefore the resultant relief was much grander. I also felt very spiritual around this point and felt like my recovery was also down to something else and that I needed to somehow acknowledge and thank it.

My job role had changed from being a PA for the managing director to now back to a more admin role. The job vacancy was called a Para planner. To be fair I wasn't happy with the shift of roles but I was so happy and so determined to stay happy that I accepted it. I had just got to a point in my career where I was going out with the MD seeing clients and getting more involved with the actual financial planning side of things, then I got unwell and kind of got demoted. I totally understand why they did it, they felt the job role was too pressurised and maybe contributed to my downfall but my job was giving me the most joy in my life.

It was around this time that a few of my Dad's friends from the pub took over a football club in Shirebrook which is near Mansfield. I'm not sure what the details were but I rang Rick the manager and said that I will be the Chairman. Typical me, I wanted to be at the top straight away without knowing anything about the club or anything about football. I was given the job as treasurer or something to that effect. Basically I pressed play on the iPod and the music came out on the PA system. I would also have a few other jobs but nothing sparkling, I think Rick had me counting shots on target and number of corners etc. But I enjoyed it as I had a purpose. One thing I did get from the club was seeing first hand how much passion there was from the community. There were many people involved and they would all love to show me there business cards even if it did say 'chief pie taster'. The area was rather deprived and the football club acted as a linchpin to the community and local economy. It made me realise how much such clubs mean to people. For a lot of them it is their life.

So now I was doing a job that I wasn't 100% happy with, whereas previously my job had become my life. Maybe in hindsight I was doing too much and possibly it did contribute to me becoming unwell but I personally don't think it did. I thought if I work hard again at my new role then I will get my old job back! This unfortunately didn't happen and I continued with the role of Para planner.

I continued with my exams and managed to pass one more exam towards my diploma after returning to work. Christmas 2010 was great as I was better so the whole family were extremely pleased with how things had panned out. I had a very low key new year, prior to Christmas I decided that I was going to have some time off from drinking as it was highlighted that my excessive drinking may have contributed to me becoming unwell, again this is a matter of opinion. So I started the New Year sober. I must admit I found it really difficult going out in social situations; I just wanted to have a drink like the rest of my friends and enjoy myself like them. I felt very out of the circle. After New Year I continued with my recovery and stayed sober, I was still just happy to be back to normal and didn't need anything else in my life to make me feel better. I started smoking again once I was better, it was kind of prize for getting my life back together. Life was just very steady, I worked and went out with my pals, I thought this was it and that I wasn't going to have anymore problems in life. I kept taking the tablets and things were good.

In June 2011 I started drinking again after roughly 6 months of not drinking. I started to drink again because I felt out of the group and I was not socialising without a drink. I think the initial feeling of being well wore of and I wanted to feel that good feeling again. My confidence was low and I turned back to my old friend. I decided I would stay off shorts so I only left the house in trousers. I drank my preferred choice of drink, John Smiths. I just needed that bit of extra something in my life, than release, something to look forward too. Drink for me gave me an immense amount of pleasure and as destructive as it can be I owe a lot to drink for the fun I had in my late teens and early twenties. My life would have been nothing without it which possibly could have been a blessing. I started drinking shandy but soon progressed from shandy to pints of beer. I said I would only have a few but eventually I was drinking copious amounts again. This was from about July 2011 through until February 2012. On my Mum's birthday in August 2011 we went up to The Yellow Lion and I was on a mission to drink as much as I could. When it was time to leave I didn't want to, I wanted to stay there and carry on. When we got back home I didn't stop drinking until every last drop of beer had gone and even then I hadn't had enough and had a couple of lagers. It was as if once I had started I just couldn't stop. I'm not sure why I did this, the feeling of being drunk was just so amazing that I would do anything to get that feeling. It felt like I was addicted to getting drunk. I wasn't an alcoholic but I just wanted to be drunk. I felt like I was the person I always wanted to be when I was drunk, that I was this great personality that everyone loved. I felt like all my demons were not around when I was drunk. At the time I thought I was very happy but in truth I was just drunk and any happiness I felt was not real. I'd drink all weekend then sober up in the early part of the week then I'd be back drinking again at the end of the week. But unfortunately it wasn't the magic cure to my problems.

We had some crazy nights in the interim period and I was spending a lot of money on drink. Some nights we were drinking 15 pints plus. I was always the quickest drinker out of the group when Vaughany wasn't around. We had too much fun really and I was heading for a fall. I think I was just getting a bit ahead of myself. I was getting too confident and cocky. In February I had a big bust up with my Mum & Dad, I said some awful things that were not true, I told my sister she would be sorry when I was gone (I was having a few interviews with a firm in Leeds and that's what I meant, my Mum interpreted as I meant if I kill myself!) I basically went off on one and I told my parents that I didn't love them and got many things of my chest which whilst drunk is not the way to do it. Anyway I woke up the following day feeling shocking and one by one the night's events came back to haunt me, slowly all the things I said were coming back to me. My Mum was upset and she told me that my Dad was really hurt with what I had said to him. I was on a massive downer and had a dreadful hangover. My parents were unhappy with how I had treated them and rightly so, I couldn't deal with the fact that I told them I didn't love them. How cruel could I be? That morning I went to Richards to sell a trailer that I had bought from him. Things went from bad to worse as this guy buying the trailer kicked up a real fuss saying I had falsely advertised it and he had driven for 2 hours. He was just about to smash my face in, so I went and fetched Richard. I agreed in the end to give this man some diesel money and he went of kicking and screaming. That was the start and end of my buying and selling career. So that just added to the bad situation. I remember when I was walking to Richard's to sell this trailer I saw a man washing his car and I thought I just want a normal life, for so long I had wanted to be something I wasn't I so badly wanted to be different. I thought in trying to be this person I'm missing out on all the normal things people do. I wanted out. I just wanted to relax and do the average things in life. So from that day in February 2012 I decided not to drink again but this time it would be for a much greater length of time. I frightened myself, how could I get so confused or angry that I told my parents that? I was 24, I wasn't 16 or 17 anymore, I had to grow up. I knew it was going to be tough but I knew if I wanted my life to progress I had to stop. Ideally I should have just reduced the amount I drank but I couldn't do that. I'm very much an all or nothing sort of guy, I either want loads of it or none at all. The problem with drinking was I found that if I just had a couple of pints then I just wanted more. Once those first pints kicked in there was no way I was going home. I don't think I ever went home early from the pub. What, go to the pub and drink 4 pints? Instead I just wanted to keep going until last orders were called and then I'd try and get a lock in. I do miss drinking but not as much as I thought, as time progresses your mind becomes less reliant upon drink, at first when I used to go out I'd think if I just had a drink I'd be much more talkative or funnier. However over time this fades and the default setting to having a drink subsides. It never totally goes. When you stop drinking you enter into a much clearer world. Its like everything is in HD and things happen you never knew existed.

26. LETS ALL GO SPINNING

I was on a no drinking mission and when I say I'm going to do something I do it, and so far I have stuck to it. Going to parties and other social events were hard but I coped, the alternative is much grimmer. So my life went on without drink and things were ok, I continued to work hard at work trying to get my old job back but there was no change. It was around this time that I started a 13 week course of Cognitive Behavioural Therapy with Claire at Swallownest Court. It was a very difficult time as I went over my whole life and tried to find reasons for my depression and psychotic episode. It was tough but looking back it was an extremely valuable exercise and still helps me now.

One of the conclusions Claire came up with was that I was a perfectionist. The problem with being a perfectionist is things are never good enough and the goals I set were unattainable. This more often than not left me feeling crushed and disappointed, what the Physiologist tried to encourage was reducing my expectations and making them more achievable. I have made progress with this although I don't think it's possible to snap out of old thinking patterns. I do however have more attainable goals about my future for instance I had the goal of being a millionaire by 30, now unless I win the lottery I know it is not possible. I look at my qualifications and current financial position and with my realistic head on I now realise that this goal is very hard to reach. I am setting myself up for failure if I don't achieve this goal, so previously with my over ambitious head on I would have been very unhappy and disappointed for not reaching these goals. The reason why I have such high goals is I read a few books and in short they all said you can have exactly what you want but you just have to focus on it. I'll let you know at 30 if they were right.

I was advised to come off the medication and that's what I did. By May 2012 I was taking no medication. The general consensus was my episode was a one of event and that I was perfectly fine. The thing with therapy is you realise you're not perfect and neither is the world. This can come as quite a shock. Especially as I felt that everything was great and my dark days were behind me. During the therapy it made me question who I was and why I act in certain ways and it highlighted to me that like everyone I have many of my own faults. I naively thought I was this really nice person but in truth I wasn't. That was a shock, I didn't want any part of me to be bad but unfortunately this is not possible. I learned the darker side of my character and why I do certain things. On the whole the exercise was very fulfilling and continues to impact my life even now.

I started doing some of my own gardening work, just cutting grass, hedges and other general gardening jobs. I was doing this at weekends and after work and was making a real go of it, I didn't have a massive amount of work on but it was enough. Some nights I would work all day at work then go out until 10pm gardening I just seemed to have an abundance of energy. I was progressing nicely, I joined a gym which I was attending 3-4 times a week and doing spinning classes there so I was in good shape both mentally and physically. Time passed and spring came and went, my gardening continued but I started to notice I wasn't quite myself. I was getting a little unhappy at work as I realised I wouldn't be getting my old job back or moving upwards anytime soon. I felt like I was just stagnant and I needed so much more from life. I remember getting very annoyed with one of the staff members for how she talked to me in an email, I asked her for a day's holiday and she said I was a pain in the neck. Its nothing now but I took such comments very badly and felt them totally unnecessary. There was a lot going on in my head and I was becoming increasingly frustrated with life. It's true when they say smile and the whole world smiles back, but I was frowning and everyone else was frowning back. My patience with Westcourt was reducing and I felt I was just going to be stuck as an administrator all my life and never actually get anywhere. In the end it just got too much for my head to cope with plus there were all sorts of other things flying round up there so I handed my notice in on 13 June 2012. I just did it totally unexpectedly and had only decided I was going to hand my notice in about 5 minutes before I went to speak to David in the boardroom. I'm not sure if you are meant to hand an actual note in or not but I didn't I just told him there and then. David sat me down and I told him, he's a very calm and collected person and gently said *'are you sure?'*. He then said was it money as he could offer me more, I said it wasn't money. Suddenly it had sunk in, I had quit my job working for a man I respected as much as anyone I knew. We talked a little in the boardroom and I realised that my real life version of the apprentice had finished. This frustrated me even more as I knew how much that job meant to me and I so badly wanted it to be different but now it wasn't ever going to be. I had made bed and had to lie in it. I remember looking on the internet at some tax tables and working out how much I needed to get by and I decided I could do it. I agreed to work a 4 week notice and then I could concentrate on my business. I had paid all of my debts of apart from the student loan so income requirements weren't so high. A short while ago I decided to invest some more money into the stock market, in true Tom style I went for the highest risk funds. I even added a few Russian securities into the mix as I had a good feeling about the Russians around that time. David thought I was crackers, he was much more cautious with his investments. That's probably why he has a lot and I have a little. These funds had returned 60%-70% last year and I was drawn in, past performance is never a prediction for future performance. I invested my entire savings which was my house deposit fund. The stocks performed ok to start with and maybe grew a few percent but then there was some concerns in Europe and the shares fell sharply. They probably dropped 20%. I hung in there and sold with a 13% deficit. I should have stopped pretending I was George Soros but I believed one day I might just get big. Until that day I will continue to fritter away my small fund pool. But you've got to be in it to win it, you'll never get a place on Wall Street without trying. After all god loves a trier. I think my mental health started to deteriorate at this point; I was under a lot of pressure. It's funny, at the time I didn't feel under pressure but now as I look back it's clear that I had a lot going on in my head. Over the course of the next few days I had progressed from just aiming to being a gardener earning a basic wage to making a fortune. I had been reading about Titus Salt and comparing myself to him (Titus Salt was an entrepreneur who made vast quantities of money in the wool industry, mainly alpaca wool, he then built a village for his workers). I thought maybe I was going to be the next Lord Sugar, I told my Grandma that I was going to call my company TAGTRAD which is Thomas Alexander Gray Trading, I didn't think anyone would realise that I was copying Lord Sugar's AMSTRAD but they did and insisted I adopted another name. A good friend of mine Alex who specialises in IT kindly set me up a website, it was a great page and I certainly owe him a favour for his efforts. His parents were having an open garden as there gardens are one of the nicest in Aston, Alex put my leaflets all around the garden so people could see them. Very kind gesture from a very good person. I was so convinced that I was going to become so wealthy that I began to question myself. I thought how am I going to act when I have so much and there are people in the world with so little. It really messed my head up, I thought I would have an overwhelming responsibility to make everyone else ok. I thought I'd start my giving away money through people's letter boxes. It really played on my mind but I looked up to the royal family and how they conduct themselves. They have a lot of wealth but still do good work throughout the world and I thought if they can do it then so can I.

27. CHANGE WAS IN THE AIR

I started to work my notice and I was becoming increasingly convinced certain people at work were not being as supportive as I hoped they would be. Now that's probably down to the fact I wasn't 100% with it and my mental health was in decline. People would say things like *'we will probably be ok without you'* and I'd take the view that they were saying something negative towards me. It's a tough one to call really but my views on things were becoming very slanted. David was giving me more and more work like back in the old days and I was helping him. I thought maybe he was doing this to show me he still needed me or maybe it was to show me what I was loosing. I'm not sure, it depends on how paranoid I'm feeling at that point as to what answer I come up with.

On 19th June 2012 I posted on Facebook

'I don't know where I'm going but I'm on my way'

This was a quote from something I read on the internet. I became very impulsive and wanted to do things there and then. I decided I wanted to go away to Spain playing golf with my Dad and brother Alex and I badgered my dad to get it booked. In the end we decided not to go to Spain as it was going to be too expensive and instead decided to go golfing in Scotland, somewhere me or Alex hadn't been before but where my Dad went when my Mum was pregnant with me, but this would be a trip that I never got chance to go on. I posted on Facebook a picture of the Whitsunday Islands with a caption

'See you on the otherside'.

I did this because I thought I was going to a better place and that place was heaven, I didn't know why I felt this but I had a strong feeling that I was going somewhere. I believed that heaven was going to be brought to my world here on earth. Often when I'm out in the fields walking on my own and the sun is shining it often crosses my mind that maybe this is Elysium. Just so easily the blue skies and turquoise oceans can vanish and the opposite can be brought upon us. The dark side. The obvious question is if this is heaven how can there be so much suffering? There's no answer to that but I believe for there to be good in the world there also needs to be bad. Just like you cannot get shade without light. Life is an equation.

It all reached a crescendo one day when I couldn't take any more from work, I went in to see Mike who was the company secretary and I told him what I thought about everything, previous to this meeting I had a lot of respect for Mike but all that went out of the window. I sat down in his office which was located next to mine on the top floor of the building. I sat down and put my feet on Mike's desk and sat back in the chair. I told Mike straight up that I was retiring and was going to play golf for a living. Mike was perplexed, as you can imagine it must have been quite frightening having a bloke stretched out in your office. Mike said how are you going to play golf with no income my reply was I will stick a flag in a field and play for free. Now Mike is a lovely bloke but I'd had enough with work, everyone was slowly sending me crazy and it was all getting a little bit picky. I thought certain people were trying to wind me up. Now in reality they probably weren't but in my head they were and I was taking no prisoners from now on. Mike offered me a biscuit and to try and frighten him more I rammed this biscuit down my throat making as much mess as possible, there were ginger biscuit crumbs everywhere. It was at this point that Mike left his office and went for back up! I quickly took my feet of the table, brushed the crumbs away under the chair and sat there like nothing had happened. Mike went and fetched David, he came in and was very nice to me. He said I think it's time we got you a taxi to which my reply was

"I think I need a limousine"

David just laughed worryingly. They rang my parents and both my Mum and Dad had to leave work and come and fetch me. I went and sat in the boardroom; Mike in his kindness went and fetched me a paper and Jean brought me a cup of tea up. My mental state was deteriorating at a fast rate of knots, by this time I thought the whole paper I was reading was related to me like what had happened in my first episode but everything had been flipped. Just by chance the front page of the paper was about a baby boy who had died in a gas explosion somewhere in the UK. Last time I was unwell there was a gas explosion in Manchester but nobody died. I believed I had given the world the warnings in 2010 but nobody listened, now a child had died. God had given us the chance to change our ways but this had been ignored and now the world would pay the price. What are the chances of the paper that day being about a gas leak? I wasn't sure what I was supposed to do but I knew, or at least thought I did, that there was something happening with someone or something. I continued to read the paper and there were other stories that I thought were there for me to see. I was left in the boardroom for another 10 minutes or so and then someone came in to tell me my Mum and Dad were here. I said bye to Matthew who was on the phone and totally ignored Jane. I made my way down the 3 flights of stairs to the entrance hall where I was greeted by my parents. On my way down I said all my goodbyes, I remember a few staff members were crying, I'm not sure exactly what they had been told. I knocked on the downstairs meeting room door and waved to Mark who was having a meeting. Mark had been a decent chap during my time at Westcourt but I felt I would always be the office junior in their eyes. I was then escorted off the premises with my Mum and Dad, I gave Jean a hug and told her I loved her for some reason, she was a lovely women but that was a little excessive. My Dad then drove my Laguna home from work as they didn't think I was fit to drive. I went home with my Mum in her car and as we drove into Sheffield my mood dropped quite considerably after what had been a crazy hour or so and I started to panic. I remember asking my Mum whether or not I was going to end up in hospital, she asked me why I thought that and then reassured me that I wouldn't. Once we were back home my mood took a sharp increase upwards again and I was back on a mission, I even went for a game of golf with my Dad later that afternoon after the whole situation at work. It was after we had finished playing golf that the thoughts of becoming a professional golfer emerged. No one knew at this stage as I kept it all to myself. I remember after we had finished playing golf my Dad's friend Alan was talking about my game and making comments about how I hit a certain shot, it was then that I thought to myself, he can be my caddy! I wasn't the greatest of golfers and probably played with a handicap of 24 at the time. So god knows why I thought I could go from that to become a professional player. But not only a professional but the greatest player that ever lived. I even went as far as to decide that I wanted to be sponsored by Versace and remember thinking how funny it would be to push a player in a pond whilst on tour. No golfers do anything like that, I was going to be an entertainer.

I probably walked out of my job in such a way because of a film I had watched a few weeks earlier, the film was called The Office. If you haven't seen it it's about a group of office workers who rebel against their bosses and screw the company over. I didn't screw the company over but took some of the films content and used it in my own life. In reality I had quit my job and had very little work on and the chances of me making a living were slim. But at the time I could only see the positive side of things, I was convinced I was the next Titus Salt or Lord Sugar and that I had a massive chance of success in business. I had read a lot of books about successful people and could see traits in their stories that I also had in my life. However my mood took a serious dip. On the 28th June, my Mum had forgotten her phone and came back from work and found me in the bathroom with the shower running but I was just stood in the middle of the room sobbing uncontrollably and I stood and hugged my mum and said I was frightened. I was crying because for the most part of my life I had tried to make other people happy, generally if other people are happy around me then I too was happy but on this day I realised that I could no longer help other people and I was heading somewhere far away and I was frightened. I had lost my direction and couldn't see where I was heading. I knew now I had to make myself happy and I wasn't sure how I was going to do that, it dawned on me that to make myself happy I would have to upset people along the way and I never had intended on acting in such a way. I always wanted both sides to win. I felt like I had abandoned my old life and was heading into unchartered waters. I spoke to my Mum for about 20 minutes and asked her to contact Adrianne at the Early Intervention Team. Adrianne was the community psychiatric nurse I was assigned to after my original support worker, Fay, left to have a baby shortly after my first episode. Both Fay and Adrianne are lovely people and helped me through some very tough times. So when I was sobbing in the bathroom I knew I needed help and that something was wrong with me. Looking back now at the whole sequence of events my mental health was deteriorating by the day, it had probably been doing so since before I left my job. At the time however you cannot see it, but close family members knew my behaviour was irrational and my parents knew I hadn't been sleeping and were very worried and they relayed this back to Adrianne. At the time I was taking a lot of over the counter sleeping tablets, far more than I should have been but still not sleeping, I just used to take one after another as my mind and body was crying out for sleep but I could never sleep. I was eating them like smarties but they didn't help one bit, once they were all gone I just lay there in a frantic state crying out for something stronger. My brain was just spinning, faster and faster.

Adrianne got me a prescription for Zopiclone which is a sleeping tablet and said she'd drop it off at home later on. My Mum texted to tell me that Adrianne had got some tablets and my response to Adrianne was

"I'm not taking any of that shit".

Then shortly after I sent that I sent another text saying

"Ok well I'll leave it up to you two as I honestly don't know what is best".

Then I sent another

"It might be a good idea that".

So as you can see my mood was all over at this point, one minute I was going to be the next Lord Sugar then I was crying my eyes out because I didn't know what to do with my life. I then wanted help and when it was offered I told them to piss off, then I changed my mind again and accepted some help. Later on that same day I phoned Richard's Dad Sammy. Earlier on in the year Richard had kindly offered to get me a shipping container to put on his land for all my gardening equipment for which I would then pay a small rent. So I rang Richard's Dad up and said Richard was up to no good and using his Dads land for his own gains, I can't for the life of me think why I did that but I was very deluded at this stage and I was trying to get my mate in trouble by being very conniving. This is a mate who at this point in my life was my closest friend. We spent a lot of time together as other mates had girlfriends and we had a great bond, he was by my side through the bad times when others drifted. Richard would always want to do things and if we weren't out drinking we'd be playing golf. He also was my main inspiration in setting my own business as I had seen the success he was having. I would always ring him when I was stuck and time after time he would drag me out of the mire, like with the trailer he sold me, he wanted me to do well. However this was the thanks I was giving him. I'm not sure why I went so against Rich, but this again proves how your mind can become infected. Richard's dad, Sammy, rang my Dad to say they were very worried about me and it was ringing alarm bells with everyone as it was so out of character. My Mum came home this day at 12:30 to check up on me and found me curled up in a ball on my bed crying uncontrollably. My blinds were down and it was all dark in my room. I was very paranoid at this point and kept looking out of the window seeing who was coming and going. I remember just lying there and was at a total loss with life, nothing made sense anymore and all my efforts to be happy were gone. I didn't know what to do, my Mum asked me to try and explain how I was feeling but I couldn't. At one point I remember her saying

"You're very lucky ...."

I said

"How can this be lucky?"

I told my Mum that Richard was working against me and didn't have my best interests at heart. I told them the he was trying to get me back drinking so that I could make a fool of myself for him to look better. This was a million miles away from the truth but it's what I genuinely thought. Once I had got all that of my chest my mood suddenly changed, I then went a little high and told my Mum that I felt great now and was off out to do some gardening jobs. By this point everybody was becoming concerned and my moods were changing by the minute let alone the hour.

I then posted on Facebook

'Only ever play a game if you are prepared to loose'.

This was a personal attack at Richard. I thought he was playing a game and it was against me.

28. WHO AM I?

On Friday 29th June I went home and gathered all the belongings that Richard had ever lent me including books, clothes, badminton rackets, golf shoes, shoes, golf clubs, DVDs, the list goes on. I gathered them all up in black bin bags and took them to his house. I just wanted everything relating to Richard out of my life. On of the DVD's was 'Secret to my success' Richard had bought it me as he had watched it and thought it reminded him of me. I thought he was taking the piss out of me and I threw it out of my car window and onto his drive when I was driving past his house on a separate occasion. I then went round to my Grandma's who lives very close to our house in Aston. I never mentioned that I had taken all the items up to Richards, we got chatting and she said that maybe I should join a golf club or do something to expand my horizons. In my eyes at this point there was nothing in my behaviour that was out of character, to me I was improving my life and getting rid of objects or people who I saw were holding me back (this despite the fact that a couple of days earlier I was in floods of tears and believed I had nothing). My Mum sent me a text to ask how I was and if I was up and about and I replied

"Hi Ma, yes I'm not too bad, just take one day at a time don't we. I'll see you later for tea, love you xxx ".

Then I went and drew £1000 out of my savings account and joined Bondhay Golf Club. It was funny when I went to join, I had a Renault Laguna car and I had just been inside joining the Club and I was on a real high and at this point, my plans to become a professional golfer were still strong and true to me. At the golf club there is a gate that you need a code in order to get out which I didn't have, so I wound down all 4 of my windows and put on tubular bells on by Mike Oldfield at the highest level, my mood now was sky high, it was just like been high on drugs, I was sharp and had no fear of anything. I went back in the clubhouse and got the code. I was rude and arrogant and didn't care about anyone. My car was outside blocking the exit and no other cars could get in or out. The sky was all very grey and the wind was howling, all the pimples on my neck were stuck up. If you listen to that song, it really has an effect on your behaviour, especially when I was in that mindset. I then wheel spun out of the car park and drove down the entrance to the club as fast as I could, still with the windows down and this very eerie song playing out. I wanted to let people know that I had arrived.

A couple of days later I remember having a panic attack when I spoke to one of my elderly clients who I did some gardening for. I suddenly thought I was getting messages from someone that this old lady was in great danger. So I called 999, I told them that this lady was in danger and they needed to get to her house immediately, once I told them that I calmed down a little bit and was become more rational. In the end I told them it was ok and that she probably wasn't in any danger at all. Something just took over my mind again and I had to act upon it.

Prior to my extravagant introduction to Bondhay Golf Club I had sent a text to everyone in my phone book inviting them to the Yellow Lion, for a launch party - I wanted to promote the launch of TAG Gardening Services or TAG Innovations as I previously wanted to use as the name. I thought about putting banners up, balloons and music. I had planned to have DJ Jean – The Launch playing as I walked in a bit like an entrance a boxer has. In the end I decided to keep it very low key and didn't do much. On the day of the party I rang Sammy (Richard's Dad) again and told him I didn't want Richard there, so Richard came to our house to see me before the launch party to wish me well and see how I was after my recent strange behaviour with him. In truth he probably wanted to knock 10 bells out of me and I can't blame him. He was more than capable of doing so, he's got some good contacts in the boxing world and certainly knows how to handle himself. My strengths unfortunately do not come in the form of physical fights. I was buzzing again and had feelings like I was high on drugs and I was an absolute dickhead when he came round, I offered him a drink and he said he would like a coffee with no sugar, I made him a tea with two sugars. We were all sat around the table in our living room as we had just had tea. We then exchanged a few words and I said I had to go get a shower as it was getting close to my big launch event. On my way upstairs I threw Richard's shoes that he'd left in our porch out onto the road. I then got into the shower and my Dad interrupted me to ask if I had seen his shoes; I just laughed and insisted I hadn't seen them. They found them after some searching and it would take me a good few months until I told him what I had done. I was fearless, the sense of power that was stored within my mind was incredible. I would have done anything to anyone to reach my goals. I made my way up to the Yellow Lion and arrived early. Earlier on I had been to Meadowhall and bought some new Levi jeans and a new shirt from Next for my little gathering and my mood was still very high. I then text my Mum

"I don't have any medical supplies! Couldn't find them at home. Can you shed any light on what is turning into a very tricky situation".

Mum replied

"They are here – no problem, why a tricky one?"

To which I replied

"No reason" (my Mum wrote down all the messages).

I had invited one of my gardening clients, Stuart, to the pub for the big launch party and he went and had a quiet word with my Dad and said he was worried about my behaviour, talking nonsense and that I was going to be a professional golfer. Now if you were to see me play golf you would understand that any ideas of becoming professional are ludicrous. I have played for a long time and I am still poor to say the least. It would be the comedy highlight of the century to see me on tour and smashing the ball straight into the crowd of spectators. When I play people ask how long I've played, I can tell in the faces they expect me to say 6 months but when I say 14 years they can't believe it. I am the only player who gets progressively worse with time and I was never any good to start with. I'm not totally sure why I still play but just like the stock market, I'm waiting for that magic day that will change our lives.

My parents had a discussion with me that night saying that not only where they concerned but other people now were starting to notice signs that I wasn't myself. I reacted very angrily at this suggestion and the idea of me being unwell. I felt threatened and went on the defensive. My Dad was telling me that I needed help from professionals; my reply was that professionals don't always know what they are doing. I referred my Dad to the 'professionals' who fitted our bathroom and that it leaked everywhere. My point wasn't great I must admit but at the time it seemed like a good one to make. I remember thinking in my head, the only professional I will be seeing is my golf coach. Before I left Westcourt I took some lessons with a very good coach called Jason. He was great, I even sent him a text asking him how long and how much money will it cost to become a scratch golfer. He must have pissed himself reading this.

My Mum, Dad and me had a blazing row that night and I was very upset and crying, the next minute once I had got it out of my system I was all smiles again.

I was starting to try and trick people to make them question their own sanity. There is a picture in our living room that was taken in Australia; it's a picture of me on a horse dressed in full cowboy clothes from my time on the station. I decided to take the picture down to see if they would notice. My Dad is into horses and used to ride a lot when he was younger and was a very good show jumper, this was up until having a very serious car accident. They didn't notice but after they had officially questioned me about my mental health I thought it was a good time to ask them where the picture was. They asked me why I had taken it down and I replied it was because I had achieved all the things my Dad wanted to do and that he was only questioning my health because he was jealous of everything I had achieved. This is not true in the slightest but just shows how poorly I was. I thought I was this amazing person that everyone wanted to be, this just shows how deluded I was becoming. This was the first night my parents had properly questioned my mental health and indicated that I needed to see someone.

I don't think I slept that night, I didn't sleep a wink for at least 2 weeks but I can't remember when my sleep stopped. On the Saturday, the day following the launch party I went to do some gardening for a woman in Sheffield. My Mum was becoming increasingly frightened and rang the Crisis Team for some advice and they told her to either take me to A & E or phone the police if they thought I was a danger, but at the time she decided to keep an eye on me and speak to the Early Intervention on Monday.

On Sunday 1st July 2012 I posted a letter that Westcourt had sent me on Facebook. It was a letter telling me that they had put me on gardening leave. I knew what gardening leave was and knew that they were being fair but I tried to make out that they were taking the piss out of me because I was on gardening leave and I had left to set up a gardening business. My mum asked me to remove it from my Facebook as our address was on it and she didn't want that out in the public domain, which I did. My friends at this point had commented to my parents that I wasn't able to hold a conversation for long and that I had told them I was going to employ two people so I could spend my time golfing. Bearing in mind at this point I didn't have many clients and would struggle to provide a living for myself. I then told them that I didn't really like gardening and was totally contradicting myself. Me and Kidder went out for tea to TGI's and I remember acting overly confident, it probably made Kidder a little uneasy. Just before he picked me up I posted a picture on Facebook with me looking a little odd with 4 crackers stuffed in my mouth. It had the caption

'I think I'm going crackers'.

That night I didn't sleep at all and was watching videos on YouTube, I would watch one video then look at others that were listed below. For instance I would listen to a Jay-Z track then click on a link to watch another. It would then go to another track which I would have never heard of. At this point I thought that my phone had been hacked by the authorities and that everything I was doing was now being watched and I was being guided in what to watch. My phone has got a camera on the front so I thought they could see my reactions when I watched something. I thought that some higher power was selecting songs for me to watch and that the links to other tracks had been pre-determined by them. I was listening to all sorts that night, one music video that stuck out that night was Jay- Z and Rihanna, it was a remix and at the time scared the living day lights out of me. I was all alone at this stage and bearing in mind I thought some higher power had infiltrated my phone this is what text came up on the video I was watching;

YOU ARE A SLAVE TO THE ILLUMINATI
YOU HAVE BEED DUPED
YOU ARE FOLLOWING DARK RELIGIONS AND YOU DON'T EVEN KNOW IT
YOU HAVE BEEN INDOCTRINED INTO THE LUCIFERIAN BELIEF SYSTEM
WE'RE GOING TO REVERSE THE SPELL
THE ILLUMINATI BELIEVE SYMBOLS GIVE THEM POWER
FEEL IT COMING IN THE AIR MASONIC SYMBOLS EVERYWHERE
I'M ADDICTED TO THE TRUTH IT'S A DANGEROUS LOVE AFFAIR
CAN'T BE SCARED WHEN IT GOES DOWN STAND FOR FREEDOM HERE AND NOW
ONLY ONE THING ON MY MIND WHO IS GOING TO FREE THIS TOWN TONIGHT?
NEW WORLD ORDER'S GOING DOWN.

As you can imagine I was now shitting myself, I thought I had been chosen to save something or someone and that there was some conspiracy theory going on and I was deeply involved. Now as I watch that video again for the first time since that Sunday night I'm not 100% sure what it's about. My interpretation at the time was that Jay-Z and Rihanna had been asked to create a video to get my attention. I thought that they were part of the Illuminati and that I had been chosen to take control of the organisation. In truth I think the video I was watching that night was in fact an anti NWO (New World Order) video but at the time I didn't get that from the video as I know very little about the Illuminati and still don't now. Instead I just created my own truth which was that I had been chosen to lead an organisation into a new era. When I was really poorly in 2010 a triangle appeared on my jeans, made up of 3 little holes. When I became better this triangle faded and just 2 holes remained. Obviously this is not possible and it was more than likely my mind playing tricks on me. Still I kept them though.

That night I was watching the videos so intently and was so focused that my heart beat was making my bed shake quite considerably, at the time I didn't have a clue was happening but I was panicking and frightened, I looked out of my window to see if anyone else had been woken up by the shaking but there was no sign that anyone else had been awoken. At this point I thought that we had had an earthquake or some small tremor of some kind. I then put on my telly and unbelievably there had been an earthquake in Japan, it wasn't a very big one but still it had been picked up by the Richter scale and had made it on the BBC news. I was convinced I had felt the earthquake from Japan so at this stage I thought I had special powers and was in some way connected to something that allowed me to use my senses to sense certain things in the world. I was so convinced that I had felt the earthquake in Japan. I put on my Facebook

'Think the earth moved for me this morning'.

My mood had now become very agitated towards my parents by this stage which was very unusual. I had organised to meet up with Adrianne and my Psychiatrist at the time, Dr Mohkter. I was becoming a little cocky and my temperament had changed considerably. I wasn't very helpful at the meeting and thought I was above them. I came away with a prescription for some more sleeping tablets. I think the doctor was quite concerned about my mental health but when my parents asked how the meeting went I just told them they thought everything was ok and that I just needed some sleep. That was a fabrication of the truth and Adrianne confirmed to my parents that I was very guarded and she had noticed a change in my behaviour. I then put 12 status updates on my Facebook including a picture of a can of Guinness, an old dirty ashtray and a picture of me when I was a pageboy aged about 4. The status read

'Good things come to those who wait'.

What I meant by this was I've quit smoking, quit drinking and will now show the world who I really am and feel success. It was also a slogan for Guinness. Plus my Mum used to say to me that good things come to those who wait.

I also put a music video on my Facebook account of Beyoncé singing the Best Thing I Never Had and tagged Richard in it. It was a music video with all the lyrics on the page. I thought all the lyrics were about my mate including 'what goes around comes back around, there was a time I thought you did everything right.' It sounds a bit silly now watching the video back but my mind had gone totally. Just after posting that video I was watching a programme on MTV and it was hosted by Hussein Bolt and I thought he was talking right at me, again similar to the music video on the Sunday night. He was listing his top 10 songs and I thought they were clues to help me with my quest. It was around this time that I text a girl called Alex, she worked at the stables that Richard and his family own. I thought at the time that I needed a partner, someone strong who could help me as I needed someone to turn to. I sent her a message saying "can I have a horse riding lesson" she never replied so I sent what I call a chaser message, and I put "how's about we exchange a horse riding lesson for a golfing lesson". She never replied again so I left it. She is very beautiful and I believed she would be great for me in my quest however it wasn't meant to be. Months later I found out that she said to Richard why's Tom sending me strange messages and was I alright. When I first saw her after those messages I feel a complete plonker.

After I got back from Australia I would go and see Richard at his equestrian stables and I would tell all the girls about my time riding horses in the outback and that I would ride for hours on end rounding cattle up. Well one Boxing Day Richard invited me out with all the girls from the stables, they put me on the an ex race horse then was prone to bucking, no actually it was the most docile horse known to man. Meet Saxon. It's what they give to people who had no hope in riding. So I the cowboy extraordinaire set of on this leisurely ride. Well I couldn't ride this horse to save my life. We headed up the road and the horse decided to start side stepping and I couldn't get the thing to change its direction. Well everyone was having a right laugh at my lack of horse riding capabilities. It had been sometime since I had been riding and I must have lost my touch a little.

My Mum and Dad were both very worried around this time and concerned with my behaviour and again rang the Crisis Team based at Swallownest Court and they were told that my behaviour was being closely monitored but nothing really changed.

Over the next couple of days I continued to be up and down and sent a few abusive emails to Westcourt demanding that they send me a cheque for £150. I had done some work and earned some commission and they never paid me. In my opinion they owed me the £150 and I wanted paying but the way I went about it was shocking. I sent them an email saying

'I would be grateful if you could send me my £150 payaway for the work I did for Mr X. This will go someone way in compensating me for wasting 4 years of my very precious life. Don't fuck with me again'.

This was a very unfair email to send, maybe it wasn't known that the money was owed to me and in fairness they probably didn't know the full story as to why the money was owed and maybe in their opinion I wasn't owed any money. I sent an email to one of the directors with a YouTube link to a video of Dire Straights performing Private Investigations and I said I was working for the FSA and had been working undercover. If you listen to the lyrics it fits in perfectly to what I was trying to say, I was trying to scare them. Westcourt and my Mum were in regular contact and they were extremely concerned about my behaviour at this point. They asked for the key I still had for the office to be returned to them immediately and ended a note to my parents with

"We hope Tom will take advice from his Crisis Team so we can get back the old Tom".

The problem was he was long gone. Mum told Adrianne about this and she advised my Mum to contact the police, Crisis Team or go to A&E. My Mum again didn't do any of these things at this stage but was realising at an alarming rate that I desperately needed professional help and urgently.

On Saturday 7th July – I was out all day on my own in my car, I told my Mum I was out golfing but instead I was just aimlessly driving around Sheffield blasting out my Best of British CD. I didn't really have any direction with life instead I was just waiting to see what would be brought my way. As I believed I was being watched I decided to walk past the Hillsborough ground where Sheffield

Wednesday play, I did this because I had put some comments on Facebook that were aimed at making people think I was taking over the club and by now my comments on Facebook were becoming increasingly odd. I believed that if I was photographed outside the stadium it would look like I had been inside to sign contracts etc. It was all getting increasingly strange but I really believed it was the truth. I sat in my car for so long in Hillsborough that my battery went flat and I had to walk to a garage to get somebody to help me.

On the Sunday I was supposed to be out for the day with my Dad at a rallying event but I decided not to go. By now I was completely against my parents and didn't want anything to do with them. I had virtually stopped all communication and had totally withdrawn myself. I posted on Facebook *"glad I've found my marbles"*. This was with a picture of my hand holding a marble. I was trying to say to everyone that I wasn't crazy. At the time I was reading a book about Economics, it was the Wealth of Nations by Adam Smith. This was a book written in the 1700's and talked about the fundamentals of Economics. I basically thought that if all politicians read some of his work then maybe we wouldn't be in the financial turmoil we are in today. On Facebook I put the Wealth on Nations book in a picture with a RAF (I served for the Royal Air Cadets) bookmark and a twenty pound note sticking out of one of the pages. The caption I put on Facebook was

"All the answers are out there you've just to open your eyes".

On £20 notes you will notice a picture of Adam Smith, I was trying to say if we listen to this chap on everyone's £20 note then we might end up getting somewhere with regards the economy. Plus its also a link to one of my favourite bands, Snow Patrol. Later on that day I had a big clear out at home and basically threw everything away – suits, shirts, ties, shoes and just left a few things in my wardrobe. I didn't think I'd need my old clothes and that I would be provided with new clothes once I got to wherever I was heading too.

On Monday morning my Mum asked me if I would like her to take all the clothes that I had packed up to the charity shop, little did I know that she wasn't throwing them out but taking them to my Grandma's for safe-keeping. I posted on Facebook *"I need a proper job"* that was a sarcastic remark as I didn't want a proper job anymore. *"Missing one marble, big reward if found"* highlighting that I probably was cracking up.

By this time my parents were updating the Crisis Team daily with my behaviour and they arranged for a meeting with the doctors and Adrianne at home but I never turned up. They told my Mum that this was typical behaviour and that they would have to call unannounced. On the Tuesday morning at 9am they arrived. There was Adrianne, Dr Mohkter and a lovely gentleman called Dave and a very kind lady called Sarah. My Mum was there and also my Uncle Mark. It was very strange when they all turned up en mass. So there I was I had finally been caught - or so they thought. We had a 90 minute meeting during which I was very argumentative and kept telling everyone there was nothing wrong with me. My Uncle Mark took me upstairs during the meeting for a quiet chat and in a kind way told me that I would probably need to take the medication. In the end I agreed to go on 20mg Citalopram and 5mg Olanzapine. I then went out for a meal for Catrina's leaving do who was a friend from school as she was moving to Scotland. We went out for an Italian in Rotherham and there were about 12 of us in total, I remember seeing on the walls *"keep your enemies close and your friends closer"* and thought I had been taken to the Italian so I could see that. They also brought out loads of puddings for free at the end and I thought it was because I was there. I thought they knew about my mafia connections. I then went home in a foul mood as I knew I would be taking the tablets and believed that by taking them I wouldn't get to where I wanted to be and that my purpose in life would never be fulfilled and the secrets I hold deep within me would be lost forever. I came in and went straight to the tablets that were on the mantelpiece, took them, glared at my parents, said I need to sleep and stormed upstairs. I was so pissed off that I had been beaten and was taking drugs again. I put on Facebook

"One day the hunted will become the hunter"

Along with a picture of me in Australia with a gun and a dead cow. I felt like I had been hunted down over the last few weeks but I was sure somehow someday I would come back fighting.

29. OUT FROM THE SHADOWS

The next day I put a picture of my Great Gran and Great Grandpa on Facebook with the caption *"just when I started to feel myself certain people want to take this away from me. Does anyone know why?"* I'm not sure why I used a picture of them but I think it's because I felt safe with them. That night I took my tablets upstairs instead of taking them downstairs, I told my Mum I had taken them but I hadn't done, instead I took them out of the packets and put them in an old DVD case. My Mum said to me *"you agreed with the doctors you would take your meds in front of us"* and asked if I would do this in future, my reply was *"fuck off"*. I was such a pleasant chap. The next day was Thursday 12th July and I put a picture on Facebook of my two empty packets of tablets, one Citalopram and the other Olanzapine. I had taken out the contents and hidden them. I put the *caption "can somebody tell me where my medication has gone? I personally blame the gypsies."* Now here I mentioned the gypsies because previously when I was having my first psychotic episode I thought the gypsies where going to take me away, this time round I thought I had the respect of the gypsy community. This is because I respected them and the way certain gypsies live and the morals they have.

The next day I had enough of taking the medication, I was working on a plot of land just in the old part of Aston where I was clearing a piece of land with my strimmer in order for them to build a house. I worked all day and my Grandma even brought her friend Ann to see me. We were all chatting and getting along fine as if nothing was the matter. While I was strimming I went over the last few weeks in my head and what was going to happen to me in the near future and realised that the next stage was not going to be easy, more casualties would be made and a serious offensive was on the cards, it was time to raise my weapons and fight for my life. I was slowly accepting that everyone in my life were no longer any use to me and that I had to break away in order to succeed with my task. I decided to have a fire to get rid of a load of rubbish on the site. The fire was quite some size and I poured loads of petrol over it and nearly lost my eyebrows when I set fire to it. When the fire started there was a massive 'bang'. As the fire was raging I decided to get in my Laguna and go and get my tablets from their secret hiding place in my drawer where I had taken them out of the boxes for the gypsy picture. I returned to the fire with both lots of tablets and proceeded to put the medication onto the fire. The medication started to melt and I took a picture of the tablets burning and posted it on Facebook along with a YouTube link to a song by Storm called Time to Burn. I left the fire roaring and went home. My good friend Sam who was working next door later told me that the massive fire burned for days. I was in close contact with Sam around this time via text and he was a good pal. Later on that day I was to have a meeting with some people from the Early Intervention Team and I remember telling a few friends beforehand that they would be taking me away. During the day I had been having numerous calls with Dave and I strongly hinted that I needed to get out of the family home. There was too much strain going on and intense conflict. I knew I had to get out one way or another. The problem was where would I go? I had no money, no job and no option.

Dave and Sarah arrived from Swallownest Court to see me, my future now was all over the place, I had gone from leaving my full time job, setting up a gardening business, thinking I was the next Lord Sugar to then thinking I was the new head of a new alliance that was going to lead the people into a new world. My mood at this point was very head strong, all communication had now ceased with my parents and I didn't want anything to do with them. I thought I was in a game and that I was just trying to survive, I thought that the Illuminati or some great force were behind me along with all the music artists that I believed were part of that organisation. But I knew they couldn't help me, I had to complete my mission on my own. Dave and Sarah stayed for about an hour, I told them point blank that I was not taking any medication and I would fight until the bitter end to make sure I would not have to take any drugs. My brother Alex came in during the meeting and told me point blank that I wasn't myself and that I needed some help, so that was another one against me. I had told Dave that I wasn't safe at home. That was extremely unfair as it wasn't true, at no time was I ever scared at home or in any danger but I knew it would get me out. If anything my parents were probably more scared of me. I was willing at this point to go into hospital as things were so bad at home. I was refusing to take my medication and my parents were at their wits end so I knew I had to get out of there. I told Dave if he couldn't get me in hospital I was moving out and going to live in Aston Hall which is a nearby hotel. God knows how I thought I was going to afford that. Anyway I agreed to go into Swallownest Court Hospital, Dave and Sarah left our house around half five. I went upstairs and got a large suitcase from up in the loft, I put all my belongings I needed in this case and packed my passport. At this point I thought Dave wasn't going to take me to hospital but instead I was going to an Airport where I was going to board a plane. I was then going to be taken somewhere, possibly

Sydney where I would be introduced to the most important asset of all. From there I would be told exactly what was going on and what on earth I was supposed to do. A couple of days previous to this I took a picture of a painting I have of Sydney harbour, a Gray's coat of arms, a Toms (shoe make) flag, 2 golf trophies I won and a box relating to my star sign, Taurus. I then put the caption *"one day maybe : ("*. I was extremely deluded at this point; in fact deluded is the understatement of the century. I came downstairs with my bag, my Mum told me not to take so much stuff as I would be home soon. As far as I was concerned I was never coming home. I sat on my own in the conservatory with my head phones on waiting for Dave to come back. So I voluntarily walked into a Psychiatric Hospital on that Thursday night, my mood was buzzing at this point, to my surprise I didn't go to the airport but actually went to the hospital. I just thought maybe they will have to allow a couple of days and soon I would be amongst the others. I was interviewed firstly by someone from one of the Teams, this was all procedure. I was claiming that I had to get out of the house because I wasn't getting on with my parents and that my safety was an issue. I insisted that there was nothing wrong with me and that I did not need any medication. I was then seen by an on-call doctor who told me that I was possibly showing the signs of a psychotic episode and that maybe a small dose of Olanzapine, he said 2.5mg, would just take the edge of things. I thought about it but I had it in my head that people were trying to silence me and that I had a message to give out so in the end I didn't agree to take any medication.

After the meeting with the doctor I was taken to my room by a lovely lady called Michelle, it turned out that I lived next door but one to her mother-in-law. That's the problem when you go to a hospital in your village, everybody knew me. Probably for the wrong reasons. So Michelle firstly went through all my items to make sure I didn't have anything I shouldn't have. She went through all my clothes and itemised them all on a sheet of paper and as I thought I was going to some sunny location to meet the girl of my dreams I packed all my best stuff! I like my clothes and I liked to spend a lot of money on clothes. So she wrote down amongst other things 2 x Dior Polo Shirts, 1 x Versace shirt, 1 x Stone Island Jumper, 1 x Burberry shirt, 1 x Boss shirt, 1 x Bellstaff coat and the list went on. She commented on my good collection of clothes and I was chuffed to bits with that. I thought it was all pre-determined and she was only doing this to boost my ego. I thought I was running the show and that everyone else was a piece in a massive game of chess. Michelle told me about what they did at night with regard to lights. When you go to bed your light is turned on every hour and staff peer at you through an observation window. You have the option to close the observation window but the staff then have to open the window from the outside with a big bunch of keys which they said will probably wake you up. I thought if someone turns this big light above my head on then I will probably wake up anyway. I went for the window open option as advised. The hospital and rooms where all very nice, I think it had recently changed from housing elderly dementia patients to an acute ward for mental health problems. The rooms had one single bed, a wardrobe, radiator and a chair. The bathroom had a toilet, shower and sink. Everything was very clean and nice bearing in mind I was in a hospital. It was all designed so you couldn't harm yourself, for example the taps were on sensors and only ran for so long, that was I guess so you couldn't drown yourself. My room was located on the female ward as all of the male rooms where taken. The female rooms looked out onto a big garden where there were lovely flower beds, bark and grass. I was fortunate to be on that section where the views where better. The male corridor looked out onto the old part of the hospital. The ward I was on was called Osprey. There are three wards in total; the other two are Sandpiper and Kingfisher. Sandpiper was a mirror image of Osprey and Kingfisher is the Intensive Care ward or more commonly down as the PICU (Psychiatric Intensive Care Unit). It was a warmish night and there were a few people in the garden area smoking and talking, I thought about going to join them but decided against it. There were also some people watching television in the lounge area but again I decided to stay in my room and listen to music on my IPhone. The track that sums this time of my life was Emili Sande's Suitcase. It was if my Mum was singing it and I thought its how she would be feeling. I listened to Emili Sande a lot around this time, the lines that caught me the most were

'You've got the words to change a nation but your biting your tongue,

You've spent a lifetime stuck I silence afraid that you will say something wrong,

If no one ever hears it how we gonna learn your song?

You've got a heart as loud as lions so why let you're your voice be tamed.

Baby were a little different there's no need to be ashamed.

You've got the light to fight the shadows so stop hiding it away.
There's no need to be afraid I'll sing with you my friend'.

Each line mirrored what was going on in my head. I had always been quiet and reserved but now I was going come out of the darkness to tell the world what I knew.

Everyday at 10pm they would call you out from your room to collect your medication, this part was like the film Cuckoo's Nest and everyone would then come from their rooms and line up ready for their tablets. In addition to receiving the medication there was also the chance to get some supper which usually consisted of toast and jam or yoghurts. So everyone would gather round the dining table to get some supper before retiring to bed. There was a tea and coffee trolley that would come out about 8 times throughout the day at various times. On the trolley were 2 flasks, one for tea and the other for coffee, after everyone had spilt milk, tea and coffee the trolley went back in until later. From memory the trolley came out at 6am, 9am, 10.30am, 12pm 3.30pm 5pm, 7pm and finally 10pm. Breakfast comprised of cereals and toast and came out between 8am-9am, lunch, which came out at 12pm, would be anything from sandwiches, fajitas, soup, baked potato or salads. Dinner was served at 5pm and was very varied from Lasagne, Roast Beef, Roast Pork, Sweet and Sour Pork, chilli, mustard chicken, chicken curry and there was always Fish on Fridays!

I however decided that I would not be eating a thing from hospital as I was convinced they were going to put Olanzapine in my food. What I did instead was get my friends to bring me takeaways, KFCs or McDonalds instead of eating hospital food. I don't know how I did it looking back but throughout my first admission I didn't eat one thing from the hospital. My first night was strange, there was a very poorly women next to my room and she would scream all night, one thing she was screaming was *"let me die, I want to die".* After hearing her loud screams I started to think what on earth had I let myself into and the reality of what I had done started to sink in. What if I'm not this important person? What will happen to me then?
The next day my Mum had sent me a message saying

"Rang the ward this morning to see how you are and thought I might pop and see you at visiting time – 3.30pm ish, let me know if ok and if you want anything bringing in xx love u xx."

My reply was

"Don't want to see anyone thank you".

My Mum then replied

"Ok babes if that's what u want, it would have been good to see you though xx seeya soon xx"

I then replied with

"Hiya Mum, I won't be seeing you and Dad for a long time, I understand you have loved me your way and brought me up your way however that way has not worked for me so far. I love you and always will do. Goodbye."

My Mum's response was

"Ok babes if that is how you feel we have to respect your wishes and we are always here for you anytime. We will always love you whatever, nothing you do will ever stop us loving you and please don't ever forget that xx".

The next day my Dad sent me a text asking how I was and I just replied *"fine".* I then sent the following to my Dad

"Please delete me out of your phone I don't ever want to speak to you again"

My Dad replied

"Why, what have I done wrong for you to do this to me"

I replied

"You will find out soon".

Now that kind of behaviour is not like me at all and I was acting totally out of character. It must have been so dreadful for their first son to be treating them that way. It makes me shudder reading it back again. I went to Nando's with Christie for tea on the Sunday night, she told my parents that I was coming over as absolutely normal to anybody who didn't know any different, but she said she could tell that I was really trying to be 'normal' but did say that I couldn't keep it up and god knows what will happen then. I remember very well going out for tea with Christie, my mind was working at 100mph and I was trying not to let my guard down, I knew one wrong move and the house of cards would fall. I was so driven and so determined that I made my mind work to the extremes so much so my mind was buzzing. I had decided that when I came out of hospital I would have to have somewhere to live so I contacted a close family friend of my Mum and Dads called Richard who I knew rented out property. He is married to Mum's best friend Rachel and we have gone on family holidays together since we were small. The flat I wanted to rent was located on a lovely estate nearby called Aston Manor (where we used to play as kids) and it was a newish property. I knew I needed somewhere to live when I came out of hospital and that moving back home was not an option. Well the flat that was local was already let out but he did tell me that he had another property but that one was located in Ranmoor. Ranmoor is one of the nicest areas in Sheffield and is located very near to the Peak District. The only problem was it was a good 30 minute drive from where all my friends and family were which when you have a car is fine but without a licence it's very isolated. I decided that I would take the flat on and move out of Aston and told him that I would rent it from him and would get onto finding out what benefits I could get to help me pay for it. Richard played an important role, not only did he help me out but also remained one of my parents closest friends during this time and although he was looking out for me he was keeping my parents informed of everything that was happening. We agreed I would take it from August as I would hopefully soon be out of hospital by then.

Prior to going into hospital I was driving my Laguna around like a mad man, I thought that my car had been set up with hidden cameras and computers in the engine so they could work out how I was driving i.e. how much I was accelerating and how much braking I was doing a bit like you see on the Formula 1 coverage where everything is monitored. I thought it had been rigged up by MI5 or some organisation relating to the Royal Family. I believed that I had to pass an extreme advanced driving test in order for them to upgrade my car. At the time I was writing messages in my phones notes to some organisation, the Illuminati or the British Government maybe. I would write things like 'did you like my driving then? I think it's about time you upgraded my car to a Ferrari, I want mine in Red and I want such and such a number plate'. I would then delete the messages so other groups couldn't see them if I was hacked. One time I drove into my old company's courtyard, I wheel spun it past the old building where I used to work and then did a 90 degree handbrake right turn and then wheel spun it out of the courtyard. It was quite good driving actually looking back, many a rally driver would have been impressed. My head was so full of chemicals that I had produced that I could focus so

Tom Gray

much and push the boundaries. Since I got better my Mum told me
that my old bosses were saying that there was a mad man
screaming up and down the car park, they said were 99% sure it
was Tom in his Black Laguna. They said if anything else happens
like this we will contact the police but I was backed up by the British
government and a whole host of famous singers so what were the
police going to do? It was like being on cloud 9, the feeling of
power was amazing, I was untouchable, laws didn't apply to me as
I was so high up in the system. Nobody was going to take this
away from me, I thought if I make one slip up then the empire I was
creating day by day would crumble and I would loose it all. I had
visions of me and Rihanna storming into my old office and
demanding my £150 that they owed me. We'd then speed of into
the sunset in my Renault listening to Tracy Chapman's Revolution.
I saw a film with Justin Timberlake in called In Time where he and a
girl take on the system and win, I thought it was going to be
something like that.

Another incident happened (before I went into hospital) when I saw
two former work colleagues, John and Matt. Apart from David, John
was probably the person I looked up too most during my time at
Westcourt this despite the fact he never spoke to me for the first 2
years. He was a very down to earth kind of guy once I got to know
him and very successful at what he did, he had a certain way about
him and you either liked him or you didn't and I guess I liked him.
Matthew was another adviser and also a nice chap, he was Mike
and Jean's son. I didn't have the same kind of relationship with
Matthew as I did with John. Before I became really unwell I did
some gardening work for John and just did some work to make his
house look a bit tidier, he was very supportive and I got to know
John a little more during my final weeks at Westcourt. Anyway I
was on my way to Dore & Totley Golf Club and it was just by
chance that I saw them both standing with their partners outside a
restaurant called Moran's which was next to the old train station in
Dore where they were celebrating somebody's 60th Birthday. So I
spun round what I'd now named on Facebook as Thunderbird 2. I
named a few of my assets after the Thunderbirds including my lawn
mower. I'm not sure why I do this but I used to love the show when
I was younger plus the fact I grew up on Tracie Island. I then went
over to the restaurant, they were stood outside next to the car park
entrance, I could drive past them and get away. That's what I did, I
put on full blast Rocket Man by Elton John and wound down all my
windows and headed towards them. I drove extremely slowly past
them with my glasses on with my hand out of the window making a
number 1 sign with my finger. This was because I thought I was
going to be the world's number 1 golfer. I then exited the

restaurant car park after redlining the Laguna and dropping the clutch. I then wheel spun all the way down Abbeydale Road with my horn on and then I went to play golf with Dave, mechanic James and my now arch enemy Richard. The game was pretty uneventful apart from Richard hitting his ball out of bounds on the first. He didn't count it on the score card as though he did. Something happened and I think I accused him of cheating on Facebook because after all that's where any golfing disagreements are sorted right? Any real man with any problem in life just heads to the book don't they? The next day after I had wrote these accusations he rang the pro up at the golf club to ask if it was out of bounds or not. It wasn't.

It crossed my mind to have the roof of my car sprayed so it was like a Union Jack that's because I thought I was some kind of funny man turned secret agent just like the Austin Power films. Shortly after all of this my licence was revoked on health grounds.

I once read an article about Robin Hood and other famous legends and decided that they were all fake and that they were a cover up. I thought there stories hid little double meanings which only certain people would understand.

So in summary, at this point I was now in training to become the head of something, I wasn't sure what but as I was very influenced by music I had visions of it being the Illuminati. That's what I wanted it to be, remember the words I showed you from that Rihanna and Jay-Z track 'Run this Town' well I thought they were trying to contact me and that was the biggest clue for me. As I said earlier, even though a year later when I re watched it, it turns out to be an anti Illuminati track (I think). But I obviously didn't know that at the time and my actual knowledge of the organisation was practically nil. I instead just made up my own future that fitted with my beliefs, dreams and wishes.

I still refused to take any medication whilst I was in hospital I thought that if I took the medication this whole fictitious world I had created would be taken from me and I would be a nobody. All my fame and fortune would be gone forever. On the 18th July 2012 whilst I was in hospital I was put under a Section 2 order due to my refusal to take medication. This meant I couldn't now leave the hospital as I had been doing. I was now an involuntary patient as apposed voluntary, it's a strange feeling knowing you cannot leave and you no longer have your freedom. However, luckily for me they still couldn't administer any drugs so I was still happy to carry on. I had my phone which at the time was my most important asset. I still had links to the outside and I could still watch YouTube. It was whilst I was under the section that I downloaded Rihanna's Talk that Talk album. After listening too it a few times I thought the whole album was about me. My first reaction after listening to the CD was she isn't shy! It was very raunchy I thought for example there is a short track called Birthday Cake which is a little explicit and basically it talks about cakes all the way through it. I love cakes so I linked the two together, I thought why else would she write a song about cake? As I'm writing this I struggle to see how I thought all her stuff was about me, it's embarrassing to think it but that was my truth at the time.

The whole album filled my body with faith, the songs were lovely and I didn't feel so alone anymore. I was gutted once the track had finished as it was like somebody had stopped talking to me. It's amazing that I could link every song to myself and what was going on in my head. How could she have done that? There are some great tracks on that album and some lovely love songs which I used to listen too in my bedroom when I was on my own. I put on this big front that I wasn't scared but deep down I was. I was just so driven to succeed that any fear was suppressed in me. I didn't have a choice, I had chosen this path and there way no turning back. It was a one way street. The days were long in hospital but I was downloading music off iTunes all the time. I downloaded Jay-Zs and Kanye West's album Watch the Throne which again I believed would give me more clues as to what was going to happen to me and where I was going. The song Illest Mother f**ker Alive rang a few bells with me as looking back maybe I was. The line

'Doctors say I'm the illest cause I'm suffering from realness'

Also meant so much to me for obvious reasons. Music was the only thing that got me through these tough times and the belief that Rihanna would at some point be my girl. Another link between me and Rihanna was the video to Take Care with Drake, the video took a long time to be made, long after the track was released. It came out just around the time all this was going on. The video has a Bull in the video and I thought they were communicating to me as my star sign is Taurus plus I was a Cowboy. In the video it shows arrows being shot at the bull and I related this to my picture on Facebook and the caption I used a few weeks prior. In fact I believed the whole song was about me, they wanted to take care of me. I didn't read any papers or look on the net as to what was actually happening in her life in the real world. Guess something inside me knew by doing so it would shatter my dreams.

So by now I was thinking Drake was in on this big quest which now is strange given current circumstances but I suppose at the time things were different. I already had his album and then I looked into other collaborations which Rihanna has done and then I'd listen to the lyrics of those. There were many reasons why I was drawn to Rihanna when I was poorly as I have discussed. It's strange as I had never really noticed her until becoming unwell. Of course I had heard her music and liked it but I didn't know who she was or what she looked like. It was far from a full blown love affair and she kind of went under the radar. It wasn't like I had her posters strewn all over the place, ok, well just a little one (not true). But after watching YouTube videos I felt connected to her, I watched an interview about how she had suffered a little and I thought with my experiences I could help her then of course there was all the stuff about the trouble she had with her partner Chris Brown. So I found all these items out and thought that I could help her and she could help me. When I was in hospital there was a magazine article that I read and it was about how Rihanna was partying a lot and drinking. I drew direct comparisons to my as I used to conduct myself in a similar way, obviously in reality she doesn't need any help but I was just creating things in my head to try and make myself feel of more importance than I actually was. I thought our two totally different worlds would come together. I posted on Facebook

"What happens when a tornado meets volcano?"

When I went to Australia in 2007 there were massive rains in the UK which led to serious floods especially in South Yorkshire and very near to where I grew up. One day when I was travelling I saw on the Australian Sky News an article about this reservoir that was about to burst its banks and there were pumps everywhere trying to prevent it from doing so as it would have flooded Whiston. It turned out that the reservoir I was watching was Ulley Reservoir which is 5 minutes from my house. Now I was at the other side of the world in Australia and I was looking at this dam where I grew up playing and fishing. Anyway about this stage I put another link in, I thought I was responsible for the rains in the UK but the floods happened when I was away so I was not in any danger, a bit like the Noah Ark story. I thought that I was meant to see the floods in the UK on the News to show me what was happening. When I left Australia there were massive floods in places that I had visited in Oz, again this was documented on Sky News and I too saw that and even the scrap yard where I took my car in Brisbane. It just so happened that Rihanna's track Umbrella was number 1 in the UK for ages whilst all of the floods were happening in South Yorkshire which my Mum was amazed at and would often tell people on numerous occasions when I got home from Oz. I of course was in Australia at the time and unaware. In the summer of 2012 the papers and news predicted serious floods and lots of rain that would be unprecedented. I posted a picture of an umbrella on Facebook and wrote something like I've got my safety gear. Have you got yours? I thought god was now going to send down the rains and commence the realignment. I was also listening to the murder *reigns* track from Ja Rule and this kind of described pretty well what was happening and also myself in many ways. Definitely worth a listen if you want to feel the connection I had with certain songs and what their lyrics meant to me.

Music was playing a major part of my life now; I was thinking that everything was about me. In hospital I appealed my section and was told that I would have to have a tribunal. One of the nurses came to my room to tell me that they had spoken to my Mum and told her that I was now under a section. The nurse then told me that my Mum seemed very concerned about me having my phone, I told the nurse that she is the one that needs locking up not me and the nurse just laughed at me.

Without the whole conspiracy theory I don't know how I would have got through those days. My freedom had now been taken away from me as I was now sectioned I didn't have a clue what was going to happen. My fait was out of my hands. All the staff on Osprey Ward were great and I built up a strong relationship with an inspirational woman call Shirley, she was the deputy ward manager. I tried tricking all the staff to make them believe I was ok and I think it's fair to say that I succeeded in doing so, other than her, she knew I was going through a manic episode and did tell my Mum that. Actually thinking about it they probably all did as they aren't daft.

Before I was sectioned I was able to come and go as I pleased; one time I went for a walk with this patient who will remain nameless. He was a very interesting character and he was totally against the system and didn't agree with medication. He kindly told me that one of the side effects of Olanzapine was death. Which I think you can agree is a serious side effect. Now this chap had been in and out of institutions for a long time. I took him for a walk as I knew the local area, we walked along this little circuit I had mapped out but he stopped off at this garden, he then proceeded to enter this garden and started to take samples from it. He pulled out some gluey parts of some Poppy plants, it turned out this was opium he told me. He said people are daft buying heroin from dealers when it's right here in your back yard. I agreed with him, he then rolled it into a cigarette and smoked it as he said it acted as a good painkiller. He offered me some but I declined. This guy was very unwell, his illness was different to mine and his future was very uncertain. In times gone by I would have naively thought that such a character had very little to offer society. He didn't work, didn't cooperate with services and generally didn't have anything to offer on the face of it. I did however give this guy my time and I got to know him. He was a gentle giant and he had some amazing ideas and views. He also told me of some of the things he had done years ago. He felt let down by the world, he didn't comply with the system and unfortunately this had had a big negative impact on his life. He would say when me and you get out of here we'll do this or we'll do that. He had so much to offer. Often the most disturbed, messed up people have the kindest hearts. Whether it be alcoholics or serious drug users. They act in this way because they are suffering and they need an escape and ultimately help. It's a similar story with people in prison, not everyone is evil in such places, of course there are incredibly evil people in there but some have something important to offer. Its not Black and White and when some smack head smashes your car window and steals your stereo for their next fix then your understanding declines somewhat. When you get these people on their own and listen to their story you will find something within them. Often the world is backwards, the well respected public figure heads often have less to offer the world than the homeless man sat in the park drinking cider. Again I'm just putting the cat amongst the pigeons, the actual truth is not so clear cut. While I was in this unique position and surrounded by all of these individuals I wanted to soak as much up as I could. One time there was this girl who was telling me how much she wanted to die and that she felt that was her only way out. I tried my hardest to say something that might just change something within her, the truth is my words probably had little impact but I so badly wanted to try and give people some light because after all I had got through a pretty messed up time before.

There was a TV/Games room in hospital right at the far end of the male corridor. In it was a TV and DVD player, one of the DVDs I had taken into hospital was the King's Speech and I'd been told that I should watch it, probably for the simple fact that it was a good film. I thought people were saying watch it because it was about me. Anyway after watching it I thought that I was going to help Prince Charles or Prince William and become their mentor and help them and other members of the Royal Family. I had always admired the Royals and thought what a fantastic duty it would be to serve them. Another film that was in the room was Happy Gilmore and as I used to play Ice Hockey and was also going to be a professional golfer I also thought that was meant for me. I believed that I would have to put on a show when I was playing on tour to entertain the crowd. The third film I watched was The Last King of Scotland which I too believed had been put there for me to watch.

I was in hospital for 13 days before my tribunal, my mood was getting higher still and by now I was completely buzzing. I thought I'd finally get my day in court where I could prove to the world that I wasn't crazy. I thought my whole life had been filmed including inside the tribunal. On the morning of the tribunal I woke up early, had a shave, well a trim as I had now grown a nice beard, and grabbed a quick shower. The showers in hospital were poor, you got 4 lots of about 1 minute blasts and they used to spray a fine mist everywhere, you know like the setting on your multi-functional hose pipe. You'd then have to get your body into a certain position in order for it to get wet. So I got ready, I put on my Great Grandpa's cricketing vest that was passed down to me after I had packed it for my big mission. I sent a picture of me in it to my Grandma on my phone saying *'look who's looking over me'*. After I had sent the picture I took off the vest and was left with my Pink striped Hugo Boss shirt and jeans. I gelled all my hair and looked the part and I was ready to show the world what I was made of. I thought that people all across the world would be sat there watching my life unfold. My tribunal was at 3pm so I had all morning to prepare. I had done a lot of research into a Psychotic episode and highlighted that I wasn't showing any of the signs of the psychotic episode which were:-

Hallucination
A hallucination is when you perceive something that does not exist in reality. Hallucinations can occur in all five of your senses:
- sight – someone with psychosis may see colours and shapes, or imaginary people or animals
- sounds – someone with psychosis may hear voices that are angry, unpleasant or sarcastic
- touch – a common psychotic hallucination is that insects are crawling on the skin
- smell – usually a strange or unpleasant smell
- taste – some people with psychosis have complained of having a constant unpleasant taste in their mouth

Delusion
A delusion is where you have an unshakeable belief in something implausible, bizarre or obviously untrue. Two examples of psychotic delusions are:

- paranoid delusion
- delusions of grandeur

Paranoid Delusion
A person with psychosis will often believe an individual or organisation is making plans to hurt or kill them. This can lead to unusual behaviour. For example, a person with psychosis may refuse to be in the same room as a mobile phone because they believe they are mind-control devices.

Delusions of grandeur
A person with psychosis may have delusions of grandeur where they believe they have some imaginary power or authority. For example, they may think they are president of a country, or have the power to bring people back from the dead.

Confusion of thought
People with psychosis often have disturbed, confused and disrupted patterns of thought. Signs of this include that:

- their speech may be rapid and constant
- the content of their speech may appear random; for example, they may switch from one topic to another mid-sentence
- their train of thought may suddenly stop, resulting in an abrupt pause in conversation or activity

Lack of insight
People experiencing a psychotic episode are often totally unaware their behaviour is in any way strange, or their delusions or hallucinations could be imaginary.

They may be capable of recognising delusional or bizarre behaviour in others, but lack the self-awareness to recognise it in themselves. For example, a person with psychosis who is being treated in a psychiatric ward may complain that all of their fellow patients are mentally unwell while they are perfectly normal.

In my opinion I only suffered from the last one and that was the lack of insight, I argued how can I have insight into something that isn't actually there. The truth was I was extremely deluded, namely paranoid delusion. In my first episode I was adamant that some organisation was going to take me away but this time I believed some organisation was going to take me away for a better life where I would become an essential part of their progression. I also was badly suffering from delusions of grandeur; I don't need to remind you of some of the stuff that was going through my head for you to know I was suffering from grandiose beliefs. I also had confusions of thought, in fact the only thing I didn't have were hallucinations. Before my tribunal I was constantly assessed in hospital I had probably one meeting everyday where the nurses interviewed me; the conversation was then recorded on a central database which the doctors could access for their own records.

On the Friday before my tribunal I created an online petition and it read as follows;

"I have been sectioned under the mental health act despite the fact the doctors and nurses cannot find anything wrong with me. The whole issue is based on my parents saying I am unwell. They themselves have not provided evidence which supports their theories that I require an intense course of powerful medication. Would somebody undergo chemotherapy treatment if cancer had not been found? The medicine they want me to go on is Olanzapine and if you look into this, carries serious side effects and the long term damage is unknown as it is a relatively new drug. All this will soon be enforced on me via injection if I do not agree to accept this.

Let's try and stop anyone else going through hell.

Many thanks, Tom Gray (that's exactly what I put and I haven't edited it, not bad for a complete fruit cake is it?)

I tried sending the petition to all my friends on Facebook but it kept freezing, this I thought would be the start of the revolution. I sent an email out to all the tabloids in the UK and I mean to all of them. I even sent emails to the New York Times and the Sydney Morning Herald but none of them replied. I was hoping for an international news story, in the letters I wrote that certain people were trying to silence me for the information I had. I was hoping for a media frenzy at the gates of Swallownest Court. I even emailed Nick Clegg, the Deputy Prime Minister, but he didn't even reply so he is off my Christmas card list. So I was getting a bit downhearted but my inner strength kept me going. I wanted to be carried out of the hospital by crowd of people all shouting and chanting my name. I wanted to kick-start a revolution against all the bad things that were going on in the world.

My iPhone played an incredible part in my life (other phones are available but they are nowhere near as good), it allowed me to access everything and even though I was locked up inside a room I could still communicate with the outside via Facebook. Even though I was struggling I felt I could share my pain with everyone on the outside and let them know how I was feeling and that all my suffering and fighting was not in vein. Of course everyone just thought I was strange but at the time I believed I was really making people think about things and question the world. It was also great to download all the music on iTunes. I had previously used a Blackberry but luckily I traded it in just before my admission. If I hadn't who knows what the consequences might have been, given the fact that I was so heavily influenced by music maybe I wouldn't have become so ill.

On the 21st July my Nannan (Dad's mum) came to visit me at the hospital, I hadn't seen her for quite a while and was able to carry on the façade. As she left she asked me if there was any message for my mum and dad and I said *"why am I here?"* She went round to see my mum and the next day my mum replied with the following text message as I wouldn't speak or see her.

"Hiya, it's mum in case I am no longer in your phone book?! You asked Nannan to ask me 'why am I here'. Unfortunately you were happy to go voluntarily to hospital rather than be treated with a minimal amount of meds to treat your relapse for a short time at home till you got back your perspective to enable you to carry on your wonderful life of work, golf, friends and enjoying yourself. Sadly you were told this on numerous occasions by your medical and psychiatric advisors, family and early intervention but you were unable to see this. For us who know you, care and love you the most in all the world we just wish you would listen to what the doctors are telling you (it's not too late) so that you can quickly get back to lead the life you choose xx we are all so sad that you are unable to see we only want what's best for you xx lots of love as always, Mum xx" (you can see where I get my writing skills from)

My short response was *"fuck you"*

A couple of days before my tribunal I had an interview with Dr Cooper in one of the interview rooms. The nursing staff who attended was Carly, she would later attend the tribunal. I think the doctor had been given some information about stuff I had been saying to people in the recent past, namely that I was going to become a professional golfer and one day the greatest player that ever lived. The doctor asked me about this and I told him straight up that I thought I could be the next Jack Nicholas. I put my argument forward and asked *"how can you knock me for being ambitious?."* I told him that you should never knock people with dreams after all, *all our dreams can come true, if we have the courage to pursue them*, well that's what Walter told me anyway. He then went on to ask me if I had any other ambitions, I told him that one day I think I will become the Prime Minister after I retire from playing golf, he asked how I would do that without having any relevant qualifications. I answered *"where there is a will there is a way"*. I was trying to prove to the world that I was perfectly sane and there I was spouting off saying I was going to be the greatest golfer then move into a career in politics. The link I had with politics was I met a nice chap in the gym called Paul and he was a member of the Liberal Democrats and regularly had visits from Nick Clegg. I thought I would get in with them and work my way up, I was going to have all famous singers and movie stars as members of Parliament. For example Plan B, I was going to have him as something important as I like the views he expresses in his music about Britain. Plus my mate Tom was going to be the Minister of State for Energy because what he doesn't know about energy isn't worth knowing and he has the capacity to solve the world energy crisis. So my kingdom as you can now see was growing and I was starting to have fingers in many pies, my plan was to slowly take over the world and create a new world that fitted in with my ideals and in short make the world a better place for everyone. When Shirley found out about my new political and sporting ambitions she took me to one side for a stern talking to, she said why on earth have you told them that? I said I was just expressing my ambitions, she thought I was playing up to the doctors and to be fair she wasn't far off. Shirley is a lovely women and a great inspiration, when she was around something deep inside me said everything will be alright. In the interview room was a phone and there was a red light on the phone, I thought they were broadcasting the interview to somebody so I was showing off.

My mood on the day of the tribunal was getting higher as my nerves kicked in, I was ready to take the gloves off and fight for my survival. I went overboard on preparation for the tribunal, I had documents coming out of my ears.

It dawned on me I was fighting an invisible war, there were no weapons but I was defending what I believed was my divine right and nobody should have the authority to take that away from me.

There are many conflicts around the world resulting in many innocent people dying but mental health issues are killing people every year from every corner of the globe, its an invisible war. The World Health Organisation estimates that there are 1 million suicides each year so over the last 50 years this equates to a serious amount of loss. Everyday families are loosing mothers, fathers, brothers and sisters. The war I was fighting didn't require weapons it required much more than that, it required courage and conviction. How many people do we have to loose before somebody listens, how many more of the true talents and geniuses have to fall before us? I just hope that in 10 years time I don't open the paper to a read about some amazing star that has left us forever. The world needs these people in it, they provide that bit of magic that everyone needs in their lives. They make us dream and grow and become something better. Yes they may be very wealthy live in big houses and appear to have everything but I guess there just like me and you. They too fight there own battles on a day to day basis and I do believe that sometimes it's even harder for them to beat their demons and rise from the deepest most darkest places. There is a reason why they are gifted with such talents, gifts often have a curse. The ATGIG (All That Glitters Isn't Gold) concept applies heavily here.

I sent my Grandma a text saying

"What are your plans/thoughts if I am deemed ok? Unlikely that may be I know. Obviously Mum and Dad are in a bad place now but have you considered how bad their place will be once I am released back into society? My Grandma's response was;

"Oh Tom, we're all in a bad place at the moment and my head hurts with thinking … whatever happens I'm sure with time and patience and lots of love we will all be able to work things out. Love to you as always, Grandmama".

I replied;

"I'm very content with the world at the moment".

My parents didn't attend the Tribunal. They sent in reports and statements to be taken into consideration. One of their arguments was that I had made some impulse purchases which of course I had. I joined the golf club which was around £750 and bought some other items. Just while we're on the subject I went to buy some top of the range Ray Bans costing £175, the extremely helpful and attractive attendant in the Sunglasses Hut Meadowhall said I could choose an additional pair as I was spending so much. I chose a nice pair of women's shades that I intended to give to Rihanna one day. The sunglasses are still in my glove box in my car, maybe one day I will find a suitable owner for these tints as they sure don't suit me. Anyway back to the tribunal. I'd made a number of big purchases and my parents were saying I was spending a lot of cash which I didn't have. Over spending is a big sign of a manic episode which was exactly what was happening. I argued that I had spent money on essentials and that I could afford it. I argued that the golf club membership was a good buy as when you worked it out it was £15 a week. I went on to say they spend much more than that on cigarettes and the point was I didn't smoke so I could afford to join the club. In my opinion at the time there was nothing amiss with my recent spending patterns. After all, the world's greatest golfer has to play somewhere.

I strolled out of my room and into the lounge to get a cup of coffee as the trolley was out; the ward was very quiet for a change. The night before I had been listening to Frank Sinatra's My Way and the song just mirrored my life totally.

And now, the end is here. And so I face the final curtain.
I'll state my case, of which I'm certain.
I travelled each and every highway.
Regrets I've had a few, but few to mention.
I did what I had to do. Yes, there were times, I'm sure you knew
when I bit off more than I could chew.
I've loved, I've laughed and cried, I've had my share of losing. And
now, as tears subside I find it all so amusing.
For what is a man, what has he got? If not himself, then he has
naught. To say the things he truly feels and not the words of one
who kneels. The record shows I took the blows and did it my way.

Yes, it was my way.

I was singing some of the words at the top of my lungs, I stirred my coffee then tapped my cup as loud as I could with the spoon. I then bellowed *'I did it my waaaaay'* and exited the living room and headed into the large gardened area that was shared with the Sandpiper Ward. The night before my tribunal I put the My Way song on my Facebook page as I wanted people to feel what I was feeling. As I exited the building one of the nursing assistants said *'do you feel better now?'* I responded with *'shut up you fat slag'* and walked out. At this point I was untouchable, no one could find anything wrong with me and I was almost certain the tribunal would see this and I would be allowed back to the outside world. I then went and sat on one of the benches and put on one of my Eminem albums. I had my feet up and I adopted a sunbathing position. I was listening to a lot of Eminem tracks and felt I could relate to him, I had downloaded his recovery album and felt a connection with him. I believed the track *Not Afraid* was written for me. Put your ear phones on and listen to that track. Bear in mind when listening to this where I'd been and where I was going. If I had a headphone socket in my head and you plugged in your earphones that *Not Afraid* would be playing very loudly. I did not fear anyone or anything the world had to offer and I was determined to proceed with my vision of taking the world forward however in reality I was locked up in hospital and had no power. I was probably up there in the garden for 10 minutes then Mick one of the nurses came up and sat with me. Mick was a lovely man, very softly spoken but very knowledgeable. I'm not sure what his views were about me but he gave me his time and offered his ideas. He didn't offer any opinion on my mental health. We had a good chat and then he left me, I then sat there and listened to some more music. The weather was good on the day of my tribunal and I was getting warm with my long sleeved shirt on. After my bit of down time I headed back into the ward and into an interview room just adjacent to the ward. This was now my nerve centre. I spread my papers out to make it look like I was doing more than I actually was. I had a booklet which for the life of me I cannot find anywhere but in it I basically slated my parents and my good mate Richard. I thought they had done things against me, I could turn any neutral action somebody might have made into a negative one where I was the victim. I made loads of notes and had a lot of paperwork. As my parents were not attending the Tribunal I had asked my good friend Matthew and my Uncle Richard (Dad's brother) to represent me. Matthew turned up just after lunch with some sandwiches, Matt was the one who I spent a lot of time with in Australia and was a good friend throughout my difficulties. Matthew would be attending the tribunal along with my Uncle Richard. After the day of the Tribunal things went extremely sour between my parents and my Uncle and still are to this day. They haven't spoken since, I know they will never forgive him for siding with me and ignoring what my parents were saying. A few days prior to my Tribunal he had been to see my Mum but hadn't told her he was going to the Tribunal and had even suggested that all this odd behaviour might be due to the fact that I was gay - I didn't know he had seen my Mum until many months after the tribunal. I've not spoken to my uncle since around September of 2012, I rang him at the end of 2012 when things weren't so good, he said he was in London and would call me back but never did. This was strange as when I was poorly he would ring me daily and visit the hospital. He then for some reason blocked me on Facebook. He was a close family member and having someone backing me up from the family was a plus for me, although why he chose to believe me after knowing my parents and our family and how close knit we all are will always remain a mystery. Both Matthew and my Uncle made statements to the hospital that were supporting my claim that I was well. The truth was I was far from ok and needed help, Matthew hadn't seen all of the information behind the scenes like Richard had. Matthew was just fighting my corner for my best interests, he had no other motives. My Grandma didn't give a statement to the tribunal but my parents had sent in a diary of my behaviour since I had left my job and began acting out of the ordinary. Facebook statuses, text messages and anything else they could think of including family history of mental health, etc, trying to fight their (which was in fact my) corner. The tribunal was supposed to start at half 2 but it ended up starting around half 3 as a massive amount of paperwork got submitted and my solicitor wanted to see it. There was a substantial amount for him to sift through and we had very limited time. He was on his own reading through all the things I had been doing and saying up too and including my time in hospital. My solicitor Peter was fantastic at his job and I couldn't have asked for anything more from him. Anyway Peter, Matt and I all sat in my nerve centre and finalised things for the tribunal. I noticed that my solicitor was a little shocked at what I had been doing and I think this made him think there was more to it than I was letting on.

Before the tribunal started I had a meeting with one of the members of the panel. It was a Psychiatrist and he was the specialist on the panel. I tried explaining to the Psychiatrist that I wasn't unwell I was just extremely spiritual and that my spirituality and positive energy was being misrepresented as having a mental health problem. I tried to explain that I was very focussed with what I wanted in life and I got the impression he understood what I was trying to say. He then left and we all headed to the tribunal suite that was located at the front of the hospital. Before we set of I had a moment on my own with Matthew and listened to All of the Lights by Kanye West. It's what a local lad called Kel comes out too when he's boxing, it got me in the fighting mood. Dr Cooper, Adrianne (my community nurse), Carly (nurse from hospital), Dave (community worker), Matthew and my Uncle Richard attended the Tribunal. I was under the impression that the whole thing was being transmitted and everybody was watching it unfold. Unfortunately I cannot discuss what happened in the Tribunal for legal reason however I was completely delirious throughout maybe down to nerves. I loved the attention, all eyes were on me and I liked that. Having so much attention being given to me added into my already manic mood. At one point I was in hysterics and they had to stop talking until it subsided. Everyone gave their evidence to the judge and his panel and we were all asked to leave while they considered their verdict. To say I was nervous was an understatement. What happens to me if they decide I am unwell and require medical treatment. What will happen to my brain then?

I will be ruined and I will never get to tell my story and the world would be sent into oblivion and I will have failed my duty. What will the repercussions of that be? Peter my solicitor came up to me and *said "Bi-Polar is a very serious illness and can create some major problems down the line"* I think he knew something was a miss. So much was going through my head, I remember trying to stare Dr Cooper out when he was giving evidence to intimidate him. He's not daft and was not in the slightest perturbed. We were all outside the court room my heart was pounding. My uncle said *"why are you talking so much?"* I replied *"if you were in my position you would be doing more than talking too much trust me."* We were told to go back into the room and we sat down. The judge delivered the verdict.

30.   JIGSAW MAN

I was freed and taken off my section. My Uncle never contacted my parents after the Tribunal. To say I was relieved was a major understatement, I was on cloud nine. I walked around like I was ten men, nobody was stopping me now. I now had to find out how I would get my girl and how I was going to get to the top. I danced back down to the ward and collected my belongings. Who's going to stop me now? I then put on Eminem's Without Me and again this mirrored how I felt at this point.

Before my tribunal I was watching loads of inspirational videos to keep my energy levels high, I was even listening to Winston Churchill speeches that he made to the country as war raged. I was fighting my own war and it was a war of good versus bad. Anybody that stood in my way was bad in my eyes – my parents, my brother Alex and one of my closest friends Richard. I started to segregate people into sections, good and bad. I also listened to King George IV's speech, Steve Jobs plus many others. These kept me going in my darkest moments in hospital. I felt I too shared the strength and determination to succeed that these inspirational people had. After I was free to leave the hospital I went to watch Matt play cricket and that night I went out with all my friends to celebrate my freedom and had a curry in Chesterfield. The night was crazy, Richard (my friend who I had alienated) attended but went home early with Kidder. Everyone in my eyes was buzzing about my release. They loved all the Facebook posts I had been putting and it felt was like we were all 18 again. I think the truth was I was just buzzing and I thought everyone else was. We were all just being daft and good old Sam was up to his usual tricks.

However while I was buzzing at my victory my family were distraught, especially my mum, dad and grandma. My Grampy and Margaret who live in Whitby had been in close contact all the time with my parents giving them love and support. They also used to ring me regularly at the hospital during my stay in the summer. Luckily for my parents they had lots of support from my Mum's side and their close friends who were there for them all the time – they didn't know what was going to happen but their gut feeling was that the worst was yet to come, they knew I was unwell and as hard as they tried once again they couldn't get the help for me.

I agreed in the tribunal to liaise with the Early Intervention Team plus any other services that were needed to help me, even though that it had been spelt out to me that I was ill I still failed to take it on board. As far as I was concerned I was perfectly ok and could carry on where I had left off. I remember seeing a member of staff from the Early Intervention Team and they were reading a book about depression, my first thought was these supposedly experts still need to read books so they obviously don't know what they're talking about. The truth was I was now extremely sick. Matthew had said that when I left hospital I could stay at his house where he was living with his younger brother. The house was on an estate called Ulley View which was coincidently the same estate I lived on when I was born. After the tribunal I felt like I had just been to court against my parents and won. The truth was nobody had won and I was the main loser I just didn't realise it at the time.

My behaviour wasn't too strange at first, friends didn't notice that I was acting differently, I was hiding my feelings very well, but deep down my illness was getting worse. I was still 100% sure that I was the earth's representative for change and had been sent by a higher power and that Rihanna was involved. By the time I'd been out of hospital for a couple of days I thought I could communicate with dead people. I was posting quirky jokes and sayings on Facebook and I thought I was getting sent messages from Oscar Wild and Shakespeare and that they helped create all the work I was doing on Facebook.

On the 26th July I sent my mum a text asking for some gardening equipment that was still in the garage at home and asked her to leave a key at my grandmas or leave one out somewhere. She replied saying she didn't want my grandma involved as a go-between as it wasn't fair to her and that they had no problems with me calling to collect my stuff. I told them I'd been advised by the Early Intervention Team not to see them alone; this wasn't true I made it up.

On the 28th July I posted on Facebook more horrendous stuff about my former employer who hadn't done anything wrong. I slated the Managing Director about the so called £150 that they owed me. I then referred to a book I had read and said 'Welcome to Hell' as I believed I had been there and now they were going to be punished for how they had treated me. I also put on Facebook references to another book I had read, both were about Thai prisons. It was 'Damage Done' I referred the title of this book towards my parents and said there was no turning back as the damage was already done. By now my illness had taken hold and my mind was running away with me, my beliefs and actions were becoming increasingly bizarre.

I arranged to meet my parents at my Grandma's house on Wednesday 1st August to discuss plans to collect my remaining belongings from home. It was a difficult meeting and the first time we had met for 3 weeks, we were all pleasant with each other but it was all very strange. I felt like I was at war against my parents. I acted all innocent and tried to make out I was the victim but in reality they were the victims, after all I was having the time of my life or at least I thought I was.

Earlier in the summer when I had agreed to take on the flat in Ranmoor it had seemed like a good idea to get away from everyone. Now I had been released from Hospital I needed to collect my belongings from my parents' house and take them to my new place in Ranmoor. The flat was very clean and tidy but was quite dated, unlike the other one nearer to Aston. The kitchen was a pale blue colour and the bathroom beige. It had a fantastic South facing balcony which looked out onto lots of trees and I had it all mapped out that when my true identity is revealed me and Rihanna would live in the very modest flat for a while sipping red bush tea while admiring the scenic beauty on the veranda. When I became wealthy I was going to do up all the flat and totally modernise it, people in years to come would be able to walk round the flat like a museum to see where the legend which of course was me, once lived. I would never own the flat but it would be worth a fortune and I was going to let Richard and Rachel have the rewards for helping me when I needed it. What a strange mind I have. I thought that the only way I was going to meet Rihanna was if I had my own place and I thought that one day she would get my address and come and see me. Just like that. One of the worlds most influential and admired artists would come see Tom Gray the village idiot from Sheffield in his 1 bedroom flat. Maybe I had watched Notting Hill too many times.

I started to move my stuff in on 2nd August. I planned it like some kind of military operation, my grandma and I would head into my Mum and Dad's at 1000 hours then I had decided that Matthew would come in as back up around 1030 hours. I remember getting up at Matt's and getting ready for the big mission to my Mum and Dad's, I got ready and headed downstairs and Matt and Tom (Matt's brother) were both still in bed. I was soon ready to leave and I remember being very apprehensive and a bit worried about going back to my parents and I had visions of my Dad being there as well and it all kicking off. Anyway in my own mind I was preparing for battle, so much so that I put on the National Anthem and went into some kind of trance and even gave a salute. I think this woke Matthew up, he thought I was watching the Olympics which had recently started on telly. But I was in preparation for battle, I didn't know who would be round at my house but I wasn't going to back down. I departed Matt's house and headed towards my parent's house. My Grandma was already there at the house. I was very cold with my Mum and didn't make much conversation. I remember the Olympics were on in the house and Jessica Ennis was on telly.

By this point I thought the whole world and everything in it was about me, not only the world but the whole universe. Of course I wasn't King, what I was instead was just some crazy messed up jigsaw man. Piecing together the wrong puzzle using the wrong pieces. The problem was all the easy straight edged pieces were running out. My theories and opinions on my involvement in the Illuminati had increased and now I thought I was going to become part of a new Royal Family but not for a specific country but for the whole world and I would be King. We would work in unison with the existing Royal Families throughout the world. I'm not too sure how I came to this view point but it was mainly down to the music I was listening to, Kanye West and Jay-Z's Watch the Throne certainly had a great impact, in one of the songs there are the following lyrics –

This is something like the holocaust, beat the odds, beat the feds, it wouldn't be wise to bet against the kid (I was the kid)

lucky lefty (I'm left handed), *I expect a 7* (my lucky number), *I went through hell I'm expecting heaven, I'm owed* (I believed I was owed money from my previous employer), *I cant be stopped, 2 seats on the 9/11, middle finger up to my old life* (that's exactly what I had done), *Graduated to the MOMA and I did this without a diploma* (I never got my diploma).

Plus Rihanna's collaboration with Coldplay Princess of China also fuelled my plans, I won't go through the whole song as I'm probably getting a bit boring with all this lyrical shite but I've got to slip one in for good measure, for example – *I could have been a princess, you'd be a king, could've had a castle and wore a ring.* When I used to listen to it I used to say *'you still can'* as I believed I was the king they were talking about. I put some videos on Facebook about the capture of Osama Bin Laden plus the 9/11 terrorist attacks. At the time I believed that somebody else was behind the 9/11 attacks and not who they wanted you to believe, I don't now. I also thought that Bin Laden was never killed and there was far more to such events than the media portrayed. I was talking about a cover up beyond belief. If I was to get my message out successfully the world as we knew it would never be the same again. I knew the impact of what I believed would be catastrophic however if the people did not find out the truth the world would be sent into perpetual darkness forever. I had been to the dark places and I felt I had been taken there for a reason. I had been shown the consequences and lived them first hand. I believed that I was going to end racism, I was going to encourage people to have children with a race different from their own, this way the next generation would all be a race of multi origin and this way all people would be more equal. At least in my mixed up mind that's what I thought. I also wanted to end war, the majority of wars are caused by religion and in my deluded mind I wanted to bring an end to this by forming a new religion and unite people bringing all faiths together. There would be no judgement based upon your religious beliefs or your colour but instead on your actions.

Coldplay's Viva La Vida sums up well who I believed I was, what my past was and where I was heading. You will be required to listen to that track around this point (you don't need to buy it just go on YouTube on your generic iPhone). I thought that DJs such as Armin Van Buren were amongst the new world and that their DJ sets where some kind of promotion of the Illuminati. They knew things that others didn't and they wanted to spread the good feeling with their work. Armin knows that when he is playing he is opening the gates and allowing people into trance heaven. I was very interested in symbols and, for example, for the Illuminati the triangle is prominent, Rihanna, Jay-Z and the Queen are all supposedly to have links with the Illuminati and Rihanna is often seen making triangle signs in her videos and live shows, the Olympic stadium had triangles all around the roof and the Queen was at the Olympics so I believed the whole games had been funded by the Illuminati plus Jay-Z, Rihanna and Coldplay performed at the closing event of the games and sang Run this Town and that was the track that kick started all my strange belief systems. I thought that stadiums where all my favourite artists play would become the new church and that people would go to see these acts perform and it would become the new place of worship, this kind of happens already. I just basically believed what people said on music tracks as the truth and thought it was about me. Also shortly before becoming unwell a friend's sister Stacy gave me a Tutankhamun table, I loved this table and decided to paint it black, I posted a picture of it along with the caption *'Everything's going Back to Black'*. Shortly after receiving the table I saw that

Rihanna and Jay-Z had a Tutankhamun figure whilst they were performing in Hackney, I put two and two together and decided that they had somehow been behind the fact that I received the table. Whilst I was out of hospital my Grandma had taken me around the gardens at Chatsworth in Derbyshire. I thought she took me so that the Duke and Duchess of Devonshire could see that I had visited their home. All the way round I was looking at things and thinking how I could make my house as grand as theirs. I thought I had a fortune lined up for me that had been building up ever since I was born. I decided I was going to base my house on the Chatsworth Estate, I was going to buy a large area of land or perhaps the Queen was going to give me a plot of land somewhere. Just like in the olden days, if you impressed the King or Queen you were given land. I decided I would build my house using the money that had been saved for me, I planned on having a large balcony where artists could perform, it was going to have lots of garden space so we could get a lot of people in to view the various acts. Just like on the Chatsworth Estate I was going to create business that not only would provide wealth for myself but by employing people it would add quality to people's lives. Of course I wanted to benefit from my great plan but what was more important to me was that the people prospered. Within the grounds I was going to create sanctuaries for people to go who were going through difficult times and needed help. I was going to create a foundation where the work carried out by me could be used all over the world and go some way in helping the people in need.

I often fantasised at what I would spend the fortune on. I started putting posts on Facebook like *'get me more gold I need gold'* then Britain would get more medals at the Olympics, I thought I was controlling everything now and it wouldn't be long until everyone knew who I was. My Facebook posts were becoming more frequent and they reached a crescendo at the beginning of August. It was around this point that I posted 82 posts in 1 hour. That's how fast my brain was working and its fair to say I put it under too much stress. Surely that must be a record for the most posts in 1 hour just using the brain? They weren't just random things they all meant something to me at the time. I believed the world was watching my every move. I tried to create a British version of Australia Day and posted something on Facebook stating that from now on there will be a British Day, I thought it was a great idea to celebrate being British, I was in Perth for Australia Day and it was such a fantastic celebration and I thought it would be great for the people of Britain to be part of such celebrations. In reality we as a nation are too frightened to create such a celebration and I feel a lot of past generations would find this very saddening.

I felt very special about my hometown Sheffield, Sheffield was once the greatest manufacturing city in the world and was renowned everywhere for its high quality craftsmen, it is still regarded as the central hub for specialist steel. Sheffield is in the middle of England, England is in the middle of the world and the world is the centre of the Universe (that is a NASA fact, I haven't made that up) this means Sheffield is the capital of the Universe and will be the main head quarters moving forwards. The greatest Olympic heptathlon comes from Sheffield as well as the greatest modern rock band, the greatest welterweight boxer, finest modern day explorer, world's finest downhill mountain biker and its home to the most magnificent national park in the world. Sheffield is the city I live in, it's the city of angels.

I was really into Ja Rule as well and especially a song called *Real Life Fantasy* as the song was about questioning what is real and what is just a dream and it fitted in perfectly with what I was thinking at the time plus Queen who are in it were one of my favourite bands when I was younger. I also watched the video and I saw little bits that I thought were put in it to give me clues and let me know that they were making the video for me. I also connected with a few of his other songs and listened to him a lot. I thought that maybe Rihanna was going to do a duet with him for me one day. Maybe that is a bridge too far.

Anyway I started to put all my belongings from my parents into Thunderbird 2, I decided that I was going to take everything with me, even the heaps of stuff hidden away in the loft. The feelings I had at this point were numb, I didn't have any love for my Mum and Dad, and my emotions had totally left me. I was that driven and motivated by my responsibilities that I had little time for anyone who stood in my way. My Grandma was amazing throughout this whole saga; she somehow stood by her daughter (my Mum) but also stood by me. She never lost her temper with me and was very understanding all of the time. I have a very close relationship with my Grandma even to this day, I'm very lucky to be surrounded by such loving people even when things became very testing. I started to load the car and my Mum bless her had got me some boxes from work, as I'm writing this I'm nearly sobbing my eyes out, I cannot for the life of me comprehend what hell I put my family through and especially my Mum. They say you hurt the people you love the most and never has a truer word been spoken. It must be bad enough seeing your kids move out but for them to move out in such awful circumstances must have been brutal. I had a few words with my Mum outside the front door and I told her this was not how I had planned things. My emotions were all mixed up but I had been brain washed and thought I was moving onto much greater things, I had lost touch with reality in the fullest sense and was now in a new world which I had created from watching videos on You Tube. We continued to move all of my belongings out of my room and into the two cars. When I had left the house to go into hospital previously I had left a load of signs, for example I had a cricket bat of my Great Granddad's and also a copy of the dictionary. When I left I put the cricket bat on top of the dictionary, my Great Granddad used to read the dictionary. So I thought I'd leave that as a little sign to say my Great Granddad was watching over my stuff. I also did the same with a flat cap of my Granddad's (my Dad's Father) which I hung on my radiator again showing to my Mum and Dad that all my stuff was been watched over. Truth be known if my Great Granddad and Granddad were alive they would have been horrified with the way I was treating their Grand Daughter and Son.

We filled both cars and I left my family home for what I thought was the last time, I didn't feel any sadness or any emotion what so ever. My Grandma and I set off in convoy from Aston to Ranmoor, it's a journey that takes about 30 minutes as it's at the opposite side of Sheffield. We arrived at my flat and started to unload the items from the two cars. I put up my picture of Sydney Harbour which I used in one of my Facebook posts. Then my Sheffield Wednesday picture went up plus a few of my photographs as I tried to make the place more homely. There was a wall in the bedroom which had exposed brick and looked very nice, apparently people had turned down the flat as they didn't like the brick effect but I loved the exposed brick. I eventually got a lovely picture of a sunset at Cable Beach, Broom pinned up and also a nice picture of Whitehaven Beach in the Whitsundays. My Grandma had bought me some other bits and bobs and soon the flat was starting to take shape. I connected up my stereo and TV and it all felt quite good, but it would be a while until I would spend my first night in the flat. When I finally unpacked all my stuff I noticed a couple of my golfing trophies had got damaged and the emblems had come off, I was convinced that my Mum & Dad had deliberately broken them when the simple explanation was they just got damaged. Lots of little things like that happened to which I attached a totally different meaning, a meaning that fitted in with my theories of the world.

As I said previously I believed that I could talk to dead people or at least have communication with them, I thought I had all of the important people who have passed over behind me, I thought they approved with what I was doing. Obviously the truth was I had no way of communicating with anyone who had died but it just exemplifies how ill I was. I believed I was being given messages in relation to what I was doing. As I had worked with the stock market I pretended on Facebook that I was controlling the price of shares for example I would say something bad about RBS and say I'm pleased that I sold all my RBS shares, then I'd say I think everyone needs to buy some shares in Lilly (who made the Olanzapine) as I think the whole world is going mad. I'd then make predictions about what the FTSE 100 was going to be in December when the world was going to end.

I just wanted it all to end and for me to get my girl, I realised around that point that I didn't want all the flash cars, big castles and lavish lifestyle I just wanted to settle down with a lovely girl and drink tea. I remember writing messages on my phone as I thought that the world was watching what I wrote, I remember writing stuff like forget the Ferrari I just want my girl, I'll be happy living in a static caravan all my life. Before I started writing this book I thought my high in the summer of 2012 was one big high, the truth be known it was a very lonely and frightening place to be. I was putting myself on the line, I thought the world was watching what I put on Facebook (due to me emailing the nations papers plus the deputy PM) so a lot of the things I was putting were very close to the point of getting locked up just for the content. They say its tough at the top and it sure was. You get to a point where your so high up that you forget what its like to be down the near the bottom. I had seen a film called 2012 and I was convinced that the world was going to end on 21.12.2012. I believed that it was going to wipe out all the evil in the world and only the good would survive and it would be me who would lead the people through the transition. If you watch the trailer for 2012 its quite something especially where there is a homeless person holding a sign reading;

REPENT THE TIME IS NOW

I even found an article online saying that the Mayan's do not predict the end of the world but instead the return of the king. This fitted into my theory that I was the original king of the world who was now back after being overthrown many lifetimes ago. What I believed was going to happen in 2012 was not necessarily a major change but instead a shift within the subconscious mind of every person on earth. They wouldn't necessarily know it but the power will be redistributed to the creators and the rightful holders, this will all be within the mind. Its like the magnetic field will change but nobody will actually see anything different. The change will be immense beyond anything known to man yet the changes will be hardly be noticed by the average citizen.

I believed that the power was going to be transferred back to the rightful owners in December. I thought that every citizen was going to fight for the right to reclaim what was there's just like I did when those foolish people at HBOS miss sold my Grandma her investment. People across the world would make a stand against these people who sold them a false dream and wiped out their savings in the name of commission. This was already in force with PPI but that was only trivial compared to what the people wanted back now. This redistribution of money would cripple the financial system, banks whose balance sheets already did not balance would not be able to cope with these new stresses put upon them. There share prices would plummet sending shockwaves throughout the global markets, banks would no longer be in a position to lend and one by one they would default and their premises would become places of worship for the new treaty. Property prices would crash as people would default on their mortgages therefore flooding the market with stock and further fuel the fire, the banks would further crumble as their collateral would simply have no value. Demand throughout the world economy would simply diminish over night, there will be no jobs as nobody will be demanding goods and services. As the banks will fall, trillions will be wiped of the globe in and the financial system as we know it will cease to exist. Money will have no value, companies will simply be worthless. Consumer confidence will fall and deflation will take hold, any wise ideas from the Fed or the Bank of England with regards fiscal stimulus would have little if any positive effect on the situation. There would only be one person who could stop the rot, it would need to be a person who not only has insight but knows the extremes of the market, the bear and the bull. The government would become bankrupt, there would be no welfare, no education and no hospitals resulting in mass riots throughout the UK, we would be in the early stages of a pandemic. We would become a major threat for terrorism due the fact we would have no defence budget and therefore no weapons to protect ourselves. We would be stripped bear and slowly but surely we would disposed of like a deceased body during a sky burial. This isn't a financial crash, recession or depression, this is systemic. The economy is like the mind, once it becomes sick it's often irreversible, we would simply rot from the inside out like a dead cow. Just like we drink, take drugs or conduct other temporary solutions to try and fix the problem the problem never gets fixed, instead you just prolong the agony but the day of reckoning eventually arrives. The economy is the same, if we don't feed the system with the right nutrients it will fail, value needs to be added and respect for the machine is essential, we must adapt a tough love strategy despite what those plant pots in the labour government believe. Sometimes tax rises and spending reductions are needed, we have the instruction guides but there just buried deep within the library collecting dust. Just like drinking, borrowing your way out of a crisis just prolongs the agony. Sometimes you just have to take the medication early and nip the problem in the bud to avoid over heating or under stimulus. Failing to do so may result in widespread use of the straight jacket.

Governments won't be able to afford the $10 Trillion US Dollars required to support the failing system. We would simply have to let the market fail and not intervene. There would only be one QE that would help us now and it wouldn't involve Mervyn buying phoney assets from the corrupt banks. Not something Mr Keynes would agree with I must admit however he did point out that in the long run we are all dead so take from that what you wish.

I had seen the way these entities treated the hard working citizens not only at HBOS but also during my time on the Pan European Cash Trading Desk at Lehman Brothers. Those who have lived by the sword will die by the sword.

I was once informed that the Halifax had a number of threats that they were concerned could damage their business and that Martin Lewis was in the top 5. Well I guess its time to re evaluate your rankings because Robyn Hood is coming back.

There will be members of the cabinet, CEO's and many other important people running around the place like headless chickens as these people only desire money and power and it will only be a matter of time when that is stripped from them. I on the other hand will be on Hamilton Island sipping Virgin Long Island Ice Tea with one of the pussycat dolls.

The problem is where will they hide? I looked once upon a time and there is nowhere.

During the time I was having these strong feelings I often listened to Vangelis' Chariots of Fire.

Change was upon us and the Power Realignment Wealth Distribution Act 2012 had commenced, you were given the warnings; 9/11, Boxing Day 2004, 7/7, Financial Crisis 2008 and the gas explosion 2010 but you didn't take the required action and now we would all pay the price.

It is important to stress at this point that these were not my actual beliefs but instead just some sick theories that my poorly mind had conjured up. It just exemplifies how far mental health sufferers can get from reality. I didn't want a financial meltdown, what would that achieve and who would benefit from such changes?

At the time I believed that I was to be in charge of the new world, which was a frightening prospect. My illness lead me to believe that I had a unique and special gift within me. I also knew that such a trait also comes with a price. Its life, you cannot have one without the other. There is always some trade and everything has a price. I had plans to separate the world into two parts, good and bad. The good people would survive and the bad people would be separated. I was going to be a fairly brutal leader. I was going to take people back to the olden days where laws and punishments were much stricter. If you committed an horrendous crime then you would be punished accordingly. So as I'm sure you can imagine this was a lot of pressure to give myself, I posted on Facebook something like 'if you think you're scared you want to try sitting where I am. Times your feelings or fear by the figure below (it was a figure of the population on earth) and you will know how I feel." (This was about the impending date in December) I truly put that much pressure on myself and took full responsibility for all of the people in the world. When I was younger I was fascinated by the predictions of Nostradamus and I was convinced he was right and that the world was going to end. There was one prediction on a certain date and I remember waiting up all night for the asteroids to hit earth and for the big wave to come. I stood right next to my door looking out of the window so when I saw it coming I could run into my Mum and Dad's room just in time to tell them how much I loved them for the very last time. Luckily that didn't happen.

My mood was changing, I'd post something on Facebook which was sombre then I'd post something which was more upbeat. My postings became extremely weird and more frequent. I posted the majority of the posts within a 2-3 day period around the beginning of August. Kidder and Vaughany had done some work at a café on Baslow Road Totley, they had supplied all the materials and worked there none stop for a good 4 days, often working through the night to get the job done. In the end the people who owned this café refused to pay my friends for the work they had carried out and also the materials therefore resulting in them loosing thousands. What I planned to do was get my suit on and conjuror up some documentation and I was going to walk into the café and explain to the owner that I was from a debt recovery company and basically just try and scare this women. I was going to make a whole host of threats which of course I wouldn't be able to carry out with the hope that my friends would receive back the money they had lost. I never got round to do this however I wish I had done it whilst I had the fury within me. I of course was going to take a cut and this would be the start of another little enterprise. The Grays.

On Sunday 5th August I arranged to play golf with Richard my good friend and two other mates called Barber David and Mechanic James. We played at Retford Golf Club and my mind was elsewhere, the game of golf was pretty uneventful apart from on the 17th green I got down and played my ball like a snooker player, it very nearly went in. My golf etiquette was none existent, I was shouting 'get in the hole' when my mates were taking their shots. I spoke very little to Richard as by now he was my archenemy and one of the main stumbling blocks to getting to where I wanted to be. On the way to the golf I was on my own and meeting the other three lads there. I was listening to a local radio station Hallam FM when the news broke that Chris Brown was getting back with Rihanna, I of course thought the whole world was about me so I thought they were playing games with me and the radio station was winding me up. I thought that there were cameras in my car so they would see my reaction, anyway I went crazy in my car, and if anyone could have seen me they would have locked me up straight away. Anyway I posted a response to the world via my Facebook account – the place where I did all my dirty laundry. By this point I had closed down all my privacy settings. Anyway I posted a silhouette of a man and a woman with a sunset background. I put something like I've decided that the true woman for me is Miss Tweedie. F**k you Ash'. I'd always liked Cheryl. I was playing games and I thought that they were too, obviously the truth was all the events were unrelated and not about me and I just looked like some crazy fool to everyone who read my posts. And a crazy deluded sick fool was exactly what I was. By this point I was feeling a lot of pressure, it was great being at the top but it was starting to become more lonely and frightening as time passed and I was no closer to getting my princess. I finished golf then I headed back to Matthew's house.

I believed that the USA series Lost had been written about me about me mainly because they had Polar Bears on a dessert island and that I had Bi-Polar. Plus one of the characters was called Loch which is a very unusual name and I too met a man called Loch when I was travelling. I felt like I was on my own little island trying to find a reason as to why I was here. These seem like trivial things now and not very significant but you can see how I could turn something unrelated and turn it back to me. I also felt like there was a purpose as to why we are all here on earth. I never watched the ending to Lost.

It was my Mum's birthday on 6th August and I sent her the following message at about 4 pm

'Happy Birthday. Where's my house warming gift you stupid slag?'

My Mum replied *'charming!!!'* to which I responded

'Yes I am charming and I have you to thank for that. I think it's time I reinstated you as a friend on Facebook. You've got a bit of bedtime reading to do, you whore'.

This is what I sent to my mum, who up until recently I loved more than anything in the world and now I was calling her names like that and it was her birthday. Who on earth did I think I was? So my behaviour was getting worse by the day, I never would have dreamt of saying anything like that if I was well. My Mum was and still is the most important person to me and I have great relationships with her and all other family members. My Facebook account was getting some use on this day and my Mum said in her notes that I put 50 plus posts on. Alex, my brother, was disgusted with my behaviour and deleted me from his Facebook account and put a status on telling everyone they needed to start telling me I was ill and challenge me as I was in desperate need of help.

Facebook floated on the stock exchange around this time and initially the share price fell. I remember thinking that Zuckerberg was trying to get everyone addicted to Facebook. But more to the point my Facebook page. Once everyone discovered who I was they would follow me incessantly. Then what was going to happen was Facebook would start charging people to use their accounts. People obviously wouldn't like this idea but they would be so addicted to it and so intrigued about what we were saying and doing that they would pay the monthly subscription. Even if Facebook only charged £1 per month per active user the Facebook Corporation would turnover £7,980,000,000 per annum which as you can see is substantial. Plus of course there would be product placing on posts etc. Who can't afford £1 per month? I wonder what would happen to the share price. What I was creating was a modern day version of the bible, this way it would all be recorded online so people would know the truth and nobody would ever be able to question the facts.

I was supposed to be going on a 4 day golfing holiday to Spain with a few lads from the pub, it had been booked since January time and I couldn't wait, as far as I was concerned nobody was getting in the way of me going on the holiday. I remember mechanic James calling to see me at Matthews's house. He came to talk to me about the holiday and my involvement. I was completely nuts by this point. I thought that the whole house I was living in was fully fitted with cameras and microphones and that when James was asking me questions my mate Richard would see my answers. James kept asking the same questions so I thought they wanted different answers so they could show people the different answers I was giving and then somebody would cut the footage so the answers I gave fitted what they wanted to hear. For example James would ask 'do you think you should go on the golfing holiday?' I'd answer with 'yes I think I should go'. He'd then say 'but we don't want you to go' so I'd answer 'well if that's the case I won't go' then he'd say 'really?' and I would reply with 'no I'm coming no matter what'. So the people behind the scenes would have a few different answers to play about with. But James and I just kept on going round and round in circles and he was getting more and more angry. He'd ask a question then I would run upstairs put my flat cap and Ray Bans on and answer him in an Irish accent. I was playing around with everyone but I think deep down I was hurting. In the end James told me point blank that nobody wanted me to go on the golfing holiday and I gave them my passport and told them to decide. I didn't believe that my friends didn't want me to go on the trip but it finally appeared I was not wanted. I told Dave at the Early Intervention Team that I would not be going then I told a friend I was still going and they would have to shred my passport to stop me boarding the plane. I then went to Meadowhall to do some shopping for my holiday as I decided I needed a man bag!! The first place I went was Hugo Boss, I felt like Julia Roberts in Pretty Woman when she goes into the shop and buys everything. I picked up about 3 t-shirts, some swimming shorts and of course a man bag! It was just hanging on a clothes rail right by the door, because I thought everything was being filmed I believed the shop heard a conversation I had had with my Grandma relating to the purchase of a man bag. It was funny how it was just lying there; it looked like it had been placed especially for me to pick it. I spent about £400 in Boss then went to Footlocker for some sneakers. I then went into Beaverbrook's and I picked up the watch of my dreams it was a Breitling Navitimer World and cost circa £6,000. I told the lady behind the counter to pull it out as I wanted to try it on, she pulled it out and I tried it on. At this point I was £150 into my overdraft and had no other money in any of my other current accounts. I told the women that I would take it. She then got it all ready, I told her that I was having problems with my card and I wanted to buy it before she spent a load of time sorting it all out. My card declined. How could the ruler of the world's card decline? I thought that I had a special card and that RBS had allowed me to buy whatever I wanted just so I continued to bank with them. I had posted something on Facebook a few weeks previous about RBS owing me £20. This was because I withdrew £20 from a cash machine and walked off and my money got sucked back in, I went into the bank to ask them if the machine showed that it was £20 up and she said it wasn't. I then took it upon myself to accuse RBS of theft and told them I was going to blow the bank up with Tomahawk Cruise Missiles. So I left Meadowhall and took all my goodies back to Matt's house including my very manly man bag but unfortunately not with my watch. I must have been at Matt's house 10 minutes when everybody turned up en mass. There was my Grandma, Matthew and my two other close friends Tom and Kidder. They were all here to hunt down the shark. Apparently Mathew had gone round to my Grandma's to ask if she would come and help as he was struggling with me, he had tried talking to me but I was adamant I was ok and didn't need to see anyone. I was in the bedroom sorting out all my purchases when I looked up and saw my Grandma. I asked her what she was doing there and she said that she'd come to help and that this behaviour had to stop now. She had taken advice from the Crisis Team and been advised to take me to Rotherham Accident & Emergency where the procedure to be admitted and sectioned had to begin. James and Tom, stayed for support and in the end all five of us went to A&E in Rotherham Hospital but as far as I was concerned there was no accident and there certainly wasn't any emergency. I went to the hospital with no challenge from myself, I knew that I couldn't control what was happening and I had a great deal of faith invested in what was happening in the world and with my big plan. I was sure that I would win somehow someday. I went to the hospital in my clothes that I was going on holiday in, I had some great new Black Adidas trainers, my new shorts complete with triangular symbols on them and a pork pie hat like Frank Sinatra wore. I was all ready for my jollies, my suitcase was all packed and as far as I was concerned I was going on that golfing holiday.

I had my aviators on too and pink socks, I looked pretty cool I must admit myself however Tom told me months later that I looked mentally ill just with the clothes I was wearing. So I was seen by the nurses and they ran a load of physical tests like they pricked my thumb, did a blood pressure test, etc, god knows what any of that lot was going to tell them. I was then interviewed by the doctors and the Crisis Team. I kept messing around, I even started playing hidey boo behind my Sinatra hat with the doctors. At this point I was feeling extremely pressured and, I was told later, started behaving quite aggressively. I had created this world where I was king and everyone was trying to pull me down, I was starting to crack but this would only be temporarily. Anyway they did all the tests and interviews and sent me on my way, I knew that things weren't looking good for me, I knew that my time in charge of the universe was starting to become heavily under threat. I had no insight into my illness and I thought everyone was working against me. So much so that by this point I had lost all contact with my parents and my good pal Richard. As far as I was concerned I wasn't going to see them again but at the time that didn't bother me too much as I was heading onto bigger and better things and there was no way I could have them in my life if I was to succeed with my ambitions of taking over the world. A good friend from school Leila sent me a message asking how I was and generally seeing if I was ok my reply was simple it read *I'm taking over the world bitch'*. That was it.

All five of us made our way back to my Grandma's house and she put on some nibbles and the lads had a few tins. I thought this is great we're all having a party, maybe there is a way of achieving my goals without losing more friends and family members. So we all sat there for 20 minutes or so then 3 people came into the house including two physiatrists. We all sat down in my Grandma's living room and I was again interviewed, I didn't tell the doctors that I was the king of the world or any other of my fantasies but unfortunately I couldn't pull the wool over their eyes. I believed that one of the doctors was Cheryl Tweedie in a body suit with full camouflage on, like they do on Ant & Dec's Saturday night takeaway where they trick people and are disguised. I have always been very fond of Cheryl. I believed that there had been a global underground competition and all performers could potentially win the ultimate prize and the prize was me and the title of princess of the world. I thought acts were trying to get me to see the truth about myself without saying it so blatantly that the general public would know. Rihanna was the greatest performer and for me and to think that a lot of her songs were about me just showed how much work she had put in, I also appreciated all the duets she had done with a lot of my favourite artists. Although I was King I did firmly believe that women would regain most power, this was confirmed in Beyoncé Run the World. I wasn't going to argue with that mob.

By this point my world was falling apart, I knew once I had some medication that my dreams and aspirations would all be shattered. My dream of getting Miss Fenty by my side would stay as some wild fantasy and would never be accomplished and my duties for the people would not be fulfilled. I was sectioned under Section 3 of the Mental Health Act, I'm quoted as saying *"I am happy to go down the mental health route as I love a good tribunal"*. The doctors said to my Grandma that usually the police would now be sent for to accompany the patient into hospital but she and my three friends said that wouldn't be necessary as they would take me there. The doctors, who my Grandma said were wonderful, told her that they had never encountered such support and friendship before. They drove me to Swallownest Court, my old stomping ground.

31. PARIS

So I was readmitted into the Sandpiper Ward at Swallownest Court on 7th August 2013 at approximately 9.30 pm that evening. I walked in through the ward doors and knew my life as I had planned was over. I knew once they got the medication in me that everything would vanish and the world would not be saved. I walked in with my head down and didn't say goodbye or turn around to my friends or Grandma who I left in the entrance hall, I held them responsible for getting me back into hospital and was very upset with them. I wasn't sure now what my future held. I was sitting down with my head on the table and my arms thrown in front of me when one of the patients came up to me and told me that he had been set up with drugs and also that a lot of bad stuff was going on in the ward. I was now becoming frightened but still kept my faith, I told myself I will survive one way or another and no matter what happens I will be ok.

When you take everything from a man and create a situation where he has nothing to loose, you inadvertently create a very powerful entity.

I can't really remember much about the first few days in hospital apart from the fact that I refused to take my medication. There was a bookstand in the hospital full of books and DVDs. This one day I went and got all the books and started to place the books in triangles using all the shelving. All the DVD titles meant something to me and it all made sense to me at the time. There was one book where it said on the back *'your past will come back to haunt you'* I went up to a patient and forced her to read out loud what was said on the book. I did this because I thought she was acting and there was nothing wrong with her and she shouldn't be in hospital. I believed there was no such thing as depression and that everyone should just get a grip and get on with their lives. This is despite the fact that I had suffered from depression very badly in the past. So by now I was on a mission and no one was going to stop me. They told me to stop but I kept going, by now I was throwing books all over. I went up to one member of staff and dropped a load of books by his feet, this was because I thought he was on the dark side and he needed to be rounded up with the rest of the people like him. Like I said before I had divided the world's population into two boxes - one good and one bad and I made the decision who went in which box. I wasn't going to hurt any of the people on the bad side but I was going to get them to build me my castle and get them to do all the labouring for the world. I thought that some staff members were going to help me but obviously they didn't, all I kept saying to myself was 'lets proceed with phase 3'. They told me that I would have to take a pill to calm down and I refused. They said "*if you don't take a pill then you will have to be forced medication with an injection*". To which I replied "*go ahead*". I thought everything was on camera including my bedroom where they took me to have my injection. I knew they wouldn't inject me and that in truth they liked my behaviour and were ready for the new world. I believed the same thing was going on throughout the world and everyone was rebelling against the evil. So I thought they were going to pretend to inject me so the people watching on the cameras (that weren't there) thought I had been injected but they didn't and they injected me. Now I didn't plan for an injection but they gave me one, they injected me straight through my triangle shorts. My mood shot down and suddenly it hit me, I couldn't believe what I was doing and what I was thinking. I was petrified now, I went from being on top of the world to being at rock bottom, I couldn't believe what I was thinking and doing. It was exactly like what happened in the 2010 episode when I took the Diazepam. This time it was the complete opposite and my world was turned upside down in a matter of minutes. My community psychiatric nurse, Adrianne, came to see me and I told her of my fears. I told her that I was extremely remorseful and didn't know what was going on in my head, she wasn't sure what to say but just assured me that I was safe now and that I would get better. It didn't help me though because I needed to be saved from imprisonment for having the ideas I was having. I couldn't believe what I had said to my mother in texts and couldn't believe the things I had said about my parents and friend on Facebook. I was disgusted and hated every part of me. I was truly petrified and couldn't see any future, all of the summers events unfolded one by one. Plus of course I hid nothing in my campaign and made my entire plan so blatant on Facebook for the world to see. I was in deep. How was I going to get out of this one then? There was no way. I agreed to see my parents as I knew I was in the wrong and I knew how much I had hurt them and craved their love. I saw them on Wednesday 8th August and I was extremely remorseful, I felt all the love rush back through my veins and I felt emotion again. The meeting with my parents went pretty well and my parents and my sister, Christie all told me that I was very poorly, I told them that I couldn't stop myself and that I felt like I was on a mission. They told me that with the right care I would soon feel better, they also assured me that they didn't have problems with me and that they all loved me. My head by this stage was well and truly fucked up. I had gone from ruler of the world to the worst person possible in the space of the time the medication took to kick in. The medication was only something to calm me down and wasn't the Anti-Psychotic that I so badly needed. The problem was the medication wore off.

The next day my behaviour reverted back to the aggressive and deluded me. My feelings and love towards my family disappeared and I was back on with my assignment, it was strange as I could feel the good side of me creep into my head but I just forced it away as I didn't want to have those emotions. My Mum came to see me on Saturday 12th August and my behaviour towards her was horrible, it was like I didn't want anything to do with her, I felt numb again and had no love for her. We sat outside and it was sunny, I had my Ray Bans on and was looking up at the sun, talking absolute rubbish and telling my mum that I wanted all my stuff out of the loft as I was looking for the final piece of the jigsaw, I'm not sure what this was and was probably just trying to wind my Mum up. I had asked Mum to bring in a bottle of Schloer to drink and it was in a glass bottle. We went into my room and I picked up the bottle and said I'd take it out to which mum replied we'll have to get some plastic cups as you can't take glass outside. I just looked at her and said

"Rules are made to be broken"

And pushed open the door and walked back outside. When visiting was over I stood up and walked back into the hospital, throwing the glass bottle high in the air and catching it, one of the nurses came over and said I'll take that Tom and put it in the recycling. I was acting totally out of character and my Mum went home and she told my Dad that she wasn't going to see me again on her own when I was acting the way I was, she was very uncomfortable and said she felt frightened, it wasn't her Tom.

Peter my solicitor came to see me and we put in for another appeal which would mean another tribunal and of course I loved a tribunal. Everyone else around me on the other hand didn't feel the same way and asked me not to bother with a tribunal but I ignored them and kept the tribunal open. My Dad came to see me that night and again my behaviour was offhand and disinterested.

My feelings and beliefs were now returning but this time they where stronger. They started me on 10mg of Olanzapine but it wasn't having any effect as yet, I didn't have a choice with regards taking the medication as I knew they would just inject me. The staff were a little concerned as I wasn't reacting to the medication as quickly as they thought. I remember thinking the thoughts I was having were not true but I soon told myself to keep on going with the deluded thoughts and I pushed the more rational thoughts away. I took another turn for the worse and slipped back into my dream world. On the night of the 11th August I took two hostages. I was waiting up all night after I refused to go to bed. The staff had been very accommodating and even made me a cup of coffee. I waited up all night and my mind was going crazy, I was having extremely strong feelings that I was some saintly person and as I've mentioned before the whole conspiracy that I had been put on this planet to save the world and make it a better place. Anyway I was having these strong feelings and something came over me like a mist - I had the most amazing sensation of power and I stormed into the operations room where the staff sat. Inside the room were a few monitors and pc's plus some white boards with information on them. So I stormed into the room and picked up a fire extinguisher and an umbrella and pointed them towards the staff. I had anger in my eyes and I knew how terrifying I could be when called upon. My sole intention was to frighten them as much as I could without physically touching them. Upon entering I locked my eyes upon a middle aged women. Also in the room was a younger man called Pete. I pointed the fire extinguisher at her face and said

"Get me a plane to Paris, I want to go to Paris"

She said

"We cannot get you a plane to Paris"

I replied

"Do you have a family?"

Again with my piercing stare, she answered *"yes"*, then I said

"I suggest you get me that plane ticket then".

They were a little startled with my entrance into their office and weren't too sure what to do. I sat myself on a chair that was free in their office. The reason I wanted to go to Paris is hard to explain but there was something within me was telling me I needed to go there. Plus in my deluded mind I believed that I would get off the plane and be greeted by all of my followers and the organisation I was working for plus of course the crown jewel. I also saw on Rihanna's website that she was touring in Japan and I wanted to get out of hospital so I could go on tour with her.

Jay-Z and Kanye West were around that time playing the track 'In Paris' around 15 times in a row in some concerts so when I heard this on the news I thought it was because they were trying to send me a message. For some reason I believed that all these people were waiting for me. The problem was I was stuck inside a Psychiatric hospital and there was no way of getting out so I knew I had to formulate a plan. The two staff members were looking a bit worried by now, the lady grabbed me and pushed me out of the office and I was just laughing in her face as she pushed me out and I just played about on the chair with my umbrella looking completely mad. So I was stuck now in the lounge area sat on a swivel chair.

The two staff members set of the panic alarm and all the lights started flashing and bells rang out, then all the staff from the other wards burst in. I was then grabbed by two big blokes and they took me into the seclusion unit. When they put me in the padded cell I shouted

"Do you know who I am? Go on my Facebook page and all will become clear".

So they chucked me into the cell. In the cell was a plastic mattress, a pot to urinate in, a bowl to shit in and some toilet roll. I thought the whole world was watching me in this cell so I put on a performance of a lifetime. If I said my behaviour in the cell was strange this would be a major understatement. I think I was at the peak of my madness; my high reached its highest on that Saturday night. I was running round the cell with the tray on my head screaming at the top of my voice *"I am Captain Cook"* as the tray looked like an old style hat. I then started to kick all the urine boxes and I was screaming *"look at me now, all you people who thought I was rubbish at football"*. I then got all the toilet roll and started throwing it around until it was all fully unwound. I kept running around the cell for hours shouting stuff as I thought the whole world was watching on big screens throughout the world. I literally didn't stop running for hours. I got to a point where I firmly believed that I was God and that I had the power to end the world or save the world. I believed that I had the ultimate power. Previous to my time in hospital I used the Mayan calendars end of the world in my Facebook postings and also used the film '2012'. I was trying to pass the word on that we were heading towards the end of the world. When I was in the cell I decided that the higher powers had brought forward the end of the world to the night I was in the seclusion unit. So I firmly believed that there was total anarchy going on around the world. In my head I gave the go ahead for someone or something to proceed with what had to be done, I gave the command. After I gave this command I sat down on the mattress and began to hum a song, it was like something you hear monks chanting - what I was trying to do was rebuild the world after it had been hit by all the various types of attacks from Mother Nature. What I was doing was trying to save the world for all the 'good' people from Armageddon.

I guess that's when I had reached my pinnacle there in the cell. I was God, although only for a short amount of time and within that time I had got rid of all the evil and left a new world for all the remaining people. Previous to my section I even posted online a video about a God Particle from the people at CERN as proof that there was a god. I'm not sure how you top being God. It takes some beating. The feeling was fantastic, the power I had within me was awesome. I had no fear of anyone or anything, as far as I was concerned, I was untouchable. I thought the whole universe was built around me and I was in the centre of everything. It's strange looking back on it how I actually believed the things I was thinking. What possibly can happen from being ok to a few months down the line believing you are God? The Psychiatrists will say it's a chemical imbalance and I agree totally but there must be more to it than that surely? But either way my mind was very powerful at this time. I stayed in the cell until about 7.30 am, I remember this as there was a clock outside the cell. They brought me a piece of toast, the sun was beaming in through the window and I was staring at the sun. So much so that when I moved away I couldn't see anything. So I closed my eyes. When I closed my eyes it left an orange mark and inside was a black mark. What it looked like to me was a silhouette of ET on a bicycle. At this point I believed there was a machine that was being used by the higher powers to put images in my head. It reminded me of the film The Matrix a bit where everyone is asleep somewhere and were all being programmed, I thought that the world was not real but instead a load of images that were being projected to create the world as we know it. It was an extremely tough time stuck in the cell as I didn't have a clue what was going to happen to me, the only thing that kept me sane (you could argue I was far from sane) but the only thing that kept me going totally crazy was Rihanna, although it was only a fantasy that had developed from a video on YouTube it certainly gave me hope when nothing else in the world did. If I knew the truth then I'm not sure what would have happened. She did however have one song on her album called Farewell and I thought she had recorded it especially for if I didn't survive what was happening to me. This Farewell track did raise concerns that potentially I wasn't going to make it through. So at approximately

7.30am a member of staff came in the room with some toast and a glass of water. I had a bite of the toast and sipped some of the water. At around 7.45am a load of staff came to remove me from the cell, there must have been around 8 of them. I was then escorted out of the seclusion unit and back to the ward however I wasn't going back to the Sandpiper ward I was going to the Psychiatric Intensive Care Unit or PICU as it was known. It was the Kingfisher Ward and I saw this movement of wards as some kind of promotion. Probably due to the fact the name had 'King' in it and I of course was the King. I half expected the SAS were going to burst into the ward and take me away and I waited and waited but unfortunately they never turned up. The Kingfisher Ward was very different to the other two wards, Sandpiper and Osprey. It only had 5 beds and was designed to be a highly intensive ward and, with my arrival, all the beds were full. The roof was high on the ward and there was some painted windows which made the environment seem rather peaceful. There was a dining area with about 3 tables in it but it was all open plan. There was a large flat screen TV on the wall with a sofa in front of it where we used to sit down and watch telly. Then behind the sofas was an operations room where the staff used to monitor the patients, some of the rooms had cameras in them where people who self-harmed were located. My room was very similar to the rooms on the other two wards however we weren't allowed any items in our rooms. Everything was very high security; we would have to go with a member of staff to the store room to get daily essentials such as toothpaste and toothbrushes. All our clothes were kept in the store rooms too and to avoid suicides we weren't allowed to have shoe laces, belts, phones, razors or earphones and all the cutlery was plastic as well as the plates. My beard grew very thick around this time. The atmosphere on the ward was very intense as all the people there including me were extremely poorly people housed in a very small space. Sparks would often fly and I found it difficult. I didn't know what would happen to me from 1 hour to the next. I got chatting to one of the guys in there and he felt he was in the system and wouldn't get out anytime soon, the other two girls were also very nice and one of them was a self-harmer. On a few occasions the staff had to burst into her room to stop her harming herself. I'm not sure if she was making attempts to end her life or she just wanted to harm herself in order to feel some kind of release. There was another guy who was fantastic, he became one of my mates whilst I was on the Intensive Care Unit and often said that we were *'Truth Wizards'*. He was a paranoid schizophrenic and had been in the system for a few months but was a really good guy and I used to enjoy being around him. The staff were amazing on the PICU ward, it turned out I knew one of the nurses through a friend, her name was Zoe and she was very kind towards me. Another nice nurse was called Grace and I used to say to myself she is my saving Grace as she was also lovely. Whilst I was inside I obviously couldn't get hold of any chocolate and the Olanzapine makes you crave stuff such as chocolate. I used to ask Grace all the time to bring me a Dime bar. Forget the impression 'you're a Dime Bar' here I was locked up in a psychiatric hospital craving Dime bars. All I wanted was to get my hands on one, Grace kindly brought me one in but it wasn't until the day I left and in the end I gave my Dime bar to one of my friends. There were some cycling machines on the ward and once I went in, I was really getting frustrated at being locked it, I felt like a caged lion. So I went on the machine and tried to push myself to my limits I felt like I wanted to make my heart explode that's how frustrated I was. I think it was just my way of venting my frustration and a cry for help.

Outside the hospital was a small garden and outdoor area however it was quite different to the other two wards as the fences were massive, there was no chance anyone would get out in a hurry. As it was summer when I was there I often sat outside and drank black coffee out of a plastic cup, nothing tastes the same out of plastic items. The food was fantastic like it was on all of the wards. The great thing about Kingfisher was they always used to have vanilla yoghurts, I could never get hold of these rare yoghurts on any of the other wards. I used to request them but they never sent them. Don't get me wrong the other yoghurts were nice but they weren't a patch on the vanilla ones. The yoghurts were from Longley Farm and were high quality ones, not some cheap crap you would expect in a hospital. When you're locked up inside it's funny how much pleasure you can derive from one yoghurt.

Just before I left Kingfisher, Dr Metta had decided to increase my dosage of Olanzapine from 10mg to 15mg, it was funny as the doctor said to me well you don't seem to be getting any better and I arrogantly said well you'll have to increase my medication then won't you thinking that they couldn't, to which he replied "that's what we will do then". It was widely said that Dr Metta makes you better. At this stage I was very much against the medication and didn't want to take it. Like I said earlier I wasn't responding very well to the medication and the doctors told this to my parents, I think it was because I so badly wanted my fantasies to be real and I used all my strength to fight normality away. Plus my mind is very powerful and I thought so hard about things that my fantasies became part of me. I was still not wanting to see my Mum and Dad whilst I was on Kingfisher, my Mum and Dad came to see me and I was very 'off-hand' with them and didn't want a lot to do with them.

When they came to see me they brought a pack of cards and my Mum said *"I'll just check the cards to make sure they were all there"* it turned out there was a king of spades missing so my Dad got a pen out and drew a king of spades on the joker. His drawing of a spade was terrible and he said *"well it will have to be a king of shovels"*. So me in my paranoid mind thought they were trying to play games with me and, as I used to do gardening, I thought they were saying you are not a king but someone who uses a shovel and also that I was a bit of a joker. There is many a true word said in jest. The upshot was I thought they were trying to make reference to the king and therefore over throw me. It's hard to explain certain things that were going on in my head, they make sense to me but for someone reading they probably don't make any sense at all. One of the nurses came in and asked if we would like a drink, my mum and dad both declined but I said

"I'll have a black coffee, half a sugar, but leave it out there they're going now"

And that was that – they were dismissed.

I remember one day asking for a copy of the Mental Health Act but I was told it's absolutely massive so instead they gave me something similar. I started reading it then I told the staff that I had found a loop hole and that I was going to be extradited to the Isle of Man as there was some ruling that stated I could. I don't think there was, I think instead I just made it up. I also took it upon myself to make a formal complaint against 4 members of staff. These staff members hadn't done anything particularly wrong, I was just feeling that way out, so I got a compliment card, completed it and posted it. I then went round all 4 patients and told them about the complaints procedure and offered to help them complete the forms. On another occasion I wrote a lengthy letter to the Chief Executive highlighting to her the fact that I shouldn't be in hospital. I was quite rude however I can't really remember what I had written which to be honest is probably a good thing. The days on Kingfisher were long however my head was so messed up that I lost all sense of time, my mind was so far in the clouds that I didn't know what it felt like to be normal anymore. I was still hoping for the fairy tale ending which was I would be rescued and taken out of the hospital. I thought that after I had contacted all the newspapers that at least someone must want to try and get me out but of course that never happened. I stayed on the ward for 10 days and then I was told that I had to move again, this time I was going back to Sandpiper. I was given all my belongings back including my laces and phone and was sent on my way. I was disappointed that I was leaving as I had built up such a strong relationship with the nurses and not just that but also with the patients. So I made my way back to Sandpiper with all my belongings, I half thought that I was going to be allowed to go home as my mind was still all over. Matthew was visiting at that particular time when I got transferred and the fact that he was there added to my ambitions of getting released. But it wasn't to be and I was moved onto Sandpiper. It was a little tricky going back as I had abused so many staff members and so many patients in the time coming up to being put in the seclusion cell plus how I acted on my previous submission on Osprey. But I wasn't going to let fear get in my way so I decided that if I was going to survive I would have to fight fire with fire and that's the attitude I took. Matthew helped carry my stuff over to my new bedroom and we started to put things in the wardrobe and drawers, etc. I still thought everything was on camera and I believed they were making me put all my stuff in the room so that certain people could see that I was still in hospital. Then I thought once all my belongings were put away that I would then be taken away and even then I still firmly believed that I was going to be whisked off somewhere where not only would I be reunited with our lass but also meet the Queen. My mood when I went back to Sandpiper was still very high, I was still very sick.

It was around this time that Matt came to see me and we were sat on one of the tables in the dining area and I aired my suspicions about Tom and Kidder, I thought they had lost their bottle and gone to the dark side with Richard and my parents (and obviously now, everyone else). I believed they were working against me. I guess at first it wasn't so clear but now the severity of my illness was showing and they couldn't go along without standing up to me. Eventually I trusted no one.

I guess the medication started to work as my strange fantasies reduced however this wasn't straight away. I remember once I was laid on my bed listening to my radio and there was some celebrity news that Rihanna had announced on Twitter that she was going to Paris on a train, this of course sent all the fans crazy as they all turned up at the train station. I in my deluded mind thought she was trying to communicate with me and letting me know she knew what was happening, after all 3 weeks or so previous I had taken my hostages and demanded a flight to Paris. Obviously now I just put it down to coincidence but at the time I had a much more different view on the news. My Grandma had bought me a portable radio so I could listen to some music in my bedroom, this wasn't allowed on the Kingfisher ward but as soon as I was on Sandpiper I took it out and I used to listen to it. I still thought all the songs were about me, for example The Script had a song out called Hall of Fame and I thought the whole song was about me, I thought they had written it for me. The song refers to *beating the world, beating the war and talking to God*. It then goes on to say *you will stand in the hall of fame and the whole world is going to know your name*. This too was the same for many other songs that fitted in with me and my mindset at the time. Another coincidental event was when I was laid on my bed and it was time for my medication and supper, I was normally up in the lounge then but this time I was in my bedroom, anyway a nursing assistant knocked on my door and shouted me to come out and get my Meds. I walked out of my room and down the corridor and into the lounge where a few people had accumulated and were watching telly. As soon as I walked through the room Rihanna came down on a swing type contraption and onto the stage, it was the Paralympics closing party and they sang Run this Town. That was the song where it kind of all started back in July. Plus Coldplay performed and they too had been very influential towards me over the years. I couldn't believe it, I was in awe and thought that the nursing staff had got me up especially so that I could watch her on telly. Again it's all coincidences but when you piece them all together you come out with a result that is so far away from the truth it is untrue. But it made me happy seeing her on telly, I was stuck in hospital and she was up there on her swing singing along oblivious to the traumas that were going on in my life. There were a few other things that happened or things that I heard on the radio that also fitted in with my theories. My Grandma was visiting me every day and she would stay until visiting times had finished. Amazing really, bearing in mind I had stopped all contact with my parents and had said such horrible things to her daughter. For the record I would never talk to my mother the way I did and call her such names, something had taken over my brain. I'm sure I've painted a pretty poor image of myself but really I'm not all that bad.

I guess that just shows the type of women my Grandma is; she just saw the bigger picture and told herself that one day things would be better. Time passed and my deluded thoughts slowly faded, my Mum came to visit me but she was with my Grandma as she didn't want to come on her own after my behaviour last time. She had kindly brought me some toothpaste but I said

'I don't need any more toothpaste as I have sufficient supplies with the 2 I have'.

I didn't really want to see her or my Dad as I was still firmly against them. The meeting didn't go too well and as Mum left I went into my bedroom and watched her walking up the path, she looked back at me and I remember pointing two fingers at my eyes and then pointing them at her – meaning *"I'm watching you"* and my Mum left feeling less happy than when she had came yet again. My Dad came to see me with my sister but again I was very off with him, I was still talking to our Christie. He was trying to talk to me and be nice and I was just ignoring him and was very cold. These were the feelings I had for another week or so. My poor Dad gave me a hug and I just stood there, I bet he felt crushed inside.

Then quite quickly all of the deluded thoughts rushed from my mind and my old self came back, the date was 1st September 2012. Now don't ask me how this happened but something happened in my brain it was as simple as that. You could argue that the medication had kicked in or you could put it down to something else, whatever it was I got the feeling of love back for my parents. As soon as I felt ok I rang my Mum up, she was shopping in John Lewis at the time and I explained that I was feeling better, that I was so sorry for my behaviour and we had a good chat. As far as she was concerned she had a glimpse that the old Tom might come back. Now when I said the old thoughts disappeared and my deluded mindset disappeared that's not totally true. I was still madly in love and still had high ambitions for myself. It's hard to explain but my feelings were so strong to me that I wanted that to be the truth more than anything in my life. I had backed up my beliefs with that much proof and used so much energy going over them in my brain that the thoughts had left scars. At times the only thing that kept me going through hospital was the fantasy life I had created. If I had known the truth and that was I wasn't going to get any of my fantasies then I'm not sure how I would have coped. Shortly after I had spoken to my Mum on the phone she came in to hospital to see me. It was just like old times, it was a sunny day and we walked outside and up to a gazebo in the garden and we got on very well and I was just myself with her, it's crazy to think that the bridges got rebuilt so quickly as a few days previous to this I didn't want to know her. My Dad came to see me also, it was a nice warm summers evening and we sat outside again, it was an amazing feeling to have and we got on great, he was telling me about all the things that had been happening over the summer whilst I was in hospital including his adventures into the world of excavation. I'm pretty sure he left our meeting feeling fantastic as I know I did after the meeting and also after the meeting with my Ma. Very close to this time Richard came to see me along with a copy of TG (Today's Golfer). Despite the horrendous things I had said to him he took it all on the chin like a real friend and accepted that I had been very poorly. We sat and chatted just like old times and the good feeling I got from that meeting remains locked inside me. I realised what a good man he was. We spoke to one of the other patients who told us stories about the Booth's (who are a scrap dealers in Rotherham) as he used to have dealings with some of them. Me and Richard listened intently to these stories as they were fascinating, afterwards we commented that these stories couldn't have been true. I guess we'll never know the answer to that one. Richard shook my hand, gave me a hug and went.

My pals agreed that they would bring in a curry for us all to eat together in the hospital. I was chuffed to bits with this as we hadn't all been together for some time and I needed some friendly faces. I didn't have any tea with the other patients as I didn't want to spoil my curry. I got us some plates and knives and forks and set the table. I was so lucking forward to seeing them plus food was really my only enjoyment whilst inside. They said they would be here at seven and seven came and no sign of them. I thought there must be a queue at the curry house or something like that. Then half past seven came and still no sign by which point I was becoming anxious and annoyed. Bearing in mind it wasn't long since the hostage debacle. Eight o'clock came and by now I was fuming, there were five plates on this table and I had to fight the urge to start throwing them around the hospital. I felt so let down. I hadn't seen them for such a long time and I felt like the kid no one picked at football. It wasn't much to ask them was it, come and see there friend who they hadn't seen for weeks and have tea with him, it might have been a nuisance to them but surely one night out of their lives wouldn't harm them. I wasn't exactly asking for one of their kidneys. I waited until nine and then ordered a pizza. The lads rocked up at half nine or so with the curry at which point I told them to get fucked off. I didn't want to see them I was disgusted. Turns out they had been in the pub all night. They say you can tell who your mates are in a crisis. Luckily the crisis was over but I'll never forget than little incident.

I was being closely watched by the nursing staff and doctors, when I started to feel better I would have regular chats with Pete (Pete was one of my hostages) and he would make notes on the system. I would also see the doctors a couple of times a week and they were monitoring my progress. My mental health continued to improve and on the 4th September I was given 2 hours escorted leave with a family member. Me, my Mum and my Grandma all went out for a drive to get a coffee at Wickersley. It was a great feeling to have my family back and for us all to get on again, my mood however was still a little on the high side but not high enough for anyone to notice, put it this way I wasn't too high that I wasn't allowed out. I still had the dreams and aspirations that I had before but they were very much watered down, I wasn't under any false pretences that I was King or had some connection to royalty. My leave was increased from two to six hours and this time I went home for the first time and had a nice proper home cooked chilli. It was an amazing feeling and that fed into my already high mood. After I had a few days with six hours leave they then allowed me to have overnight leave over the weekend. This was great, the beds in hospital were so hard it was untrue. My bed at home was like heaven, it was so comfy. My head however was still all over the place and I found sleeping very tough. So much so that they prescribed me some Zopiclone to try and help me with my sleeping. They worked to some extent but they didn't solve the problem. Previously when I moved out in August I told my brother Alex to move into my room, the main reason I did this was to spite my Mum, for some reason I thought it might annoy her. So when I came home I was in the attic which used to be my brothers. My brother also had some important news over the summer whilst I was very unwell that he and his partner Nicole would be having their first child, this meant our family would have 5 generations as my Great-Gran is still alive.

So I gradually moved out of hospital and back home, on the surface I appeared to be ok but I was still having some strange thoughts and my plan was still there but had been suppressed massively. The light of my high was slowly fading but it wasn't out and I was clinging on to it with all my strength.

I was still posting things on Facebook and I thought my Facebook campaign was still going, for instance I put a link to the Run This Town video along with the caption 'we're not running this town' which is a strange thing to put, my entire friends list on Facebook must think I am the most bizarre person on their contacts. I began more and more to come of my high and I was discharged from my section on 24th September 2012 which I had been on for roughly 12 weeks in total, less of course the time period between winning my tribunal and my section 3 (1 week or so). Plus there were the weeks before I was put under a section 2 when I first went voluntarily into hospital which was approximately 2 weeks. I still wasn't myself but given the past few months I had endured that wasn't really much of a surprise. Things at first were fine at home, my mood was a little high in the early days but over time it came down to a more normal level. I was probably fine for about 8 weeks after being discharged and my mood levelled out and became at a more normal level and life kind of felt normal. I was ok for September and October but I started to have major concerns about what I had put on Facebook during the summer months and what I had said to my family. The high was well and truly over.

32. KARMA HOTEL

It was like the hangover from hell. I suppose it was my body's way of adjusting and was inevitable, I guess if you go out drinking for three days then the days after you stop are rough but when you go on a bender for 3 months you have to accept things are going to be a bit more shitty. Maybe that or maybe it was Gods way of punishing me for trying to wage such terror upon his people. Maybe I was just some greedy power driven idiot trying to find fame and fortune by fabricating a whole theory based on my own sick ideals. I know the answer to that but I'm not going to tell you. During October I decided I felt well enough to move into the flat I was still renting but of course hadn't lived in yet due to me been put under a section 3 resulting in my incarceration at Swallownest Court. I went on a shopping expedition to IKEA in Nottingham with my Mum and Grandma and bought all bits and bobs for the flat including a mini ironing board which rests on your legs which I thought was very innovative. When I took the flat on I was in a strange place, a place where I wanted to disappear so no one knew where I was and I could just sit alone but after getting discharged I wanted to be around my family more. I still wasn't allowed to drive and my flat was at the other side of Sheffield so I would go and stay there for a couple of days and then come home. This continued for a month or so but I was finding it tough being at the other end of town when my friends and family were miles away, especially without my car. When I moved into my new flat I used to spend a lot of time just sat around listening to the radio and looking at the birds and squirrels that used to jump about in the trees like monkeys. The scenery from my flat was immense, even Bill Oddie would have liked it. I would only go for a couple of days at a time then come back to Aston and stay there. I had no purpose in life, I just used to do things to try and make the day go quicker. I was starting to find little enjoyment in anything and just counted down time until I could go to bed. It was around this time that Rihanna released her Diamonds song, a lot of me wanted to believe that this song was about me deep down I knew it wasn't. I clung on to that fantasy for as long as I could then it left me for good. I sat in my room waiting for her to knock on my door but the doorbell never rang. After my fantasies had come to an end I was left with nothing. I was a 25 year old man from Sheffield who had quit his job, lost the plot and ended up in a psychiatric hospital. I didn't have a partner which after the summer's beliefs was a bitter pill to swallow. The truth hit me like a ton of bricks, my fantasy world was almost finished with the dreams and aspirations of improving the world were all but vanished. It was like my identity had gone, I was falling from a high place and I didn't have anything to land on. They say its tough at the top, that I agree, but the fall back down is even harder.

I felt very alone in my flat but I was trying my best to beat it, I didn't have a great deal to get up for so I used to stay in bed until 2pm some afternoons, I'd then make an effort and walk to a nearby area called Broomhill but I just didn't feel right. I had always liked the idea of living in Ranmoor as it was one of the most affluent areas and it was very nice but I wasn't from there and my life was back home in Aston. I think it would have been hard enough to move to a new part of town but coupled into the fact I had been in hospital all summer and I had an illness to contend with it made life that little bit more difficult. I didn't do much cooking and was fairly lazy, I tended to have microwave meals but did some cooking on occasions. I used to beat myself up about being lazy due to the fact I stayed in bed so long and didn't cook. I probably should have been much kinder to myself and realised that I wasn't going to be firing on all cylinders. I think my Mum and Dad realised the flat wasn't working out for me and said it was no problem if I wanted to move back home until I got myself sorted out. I stayed at the flat until the early November at which point I spoke with the Landlord, Richard and he let me practically move out straight away. I hoped that by moving back home it would make me feel a bit better about myself, I guess in truth it did a little but that was short lived and my general outlook on life took another dip. I decided I needed to get a job and get some purpose back in my life and some good friends of my parents, Rick and Jo asked if I wanted to do some voluntary work on a calendar stall in a nearby shopping centre called Crystal Peaks. At first it was great and I really got into it however over the next few weeks my mood was to take a major nosedive. There was something within me that was telling me something very bad was going to happen.

As a family we used to watch the X-Factor religiously on a Saturday and Sunday night and I was dreading the night when Rihanna would perform live to the nation as I would have to sit with everyone and watch it. Each week when they announced who was on and it wasn't her I thought thank god for that. They all knew from my Facebook posts about the feelings I had for her when I was unwell and I found all the things I had said and thought very embarrassing and difficult. Anyway the night came and she performed Diamonds in a shower, it was hard seeing the girl of your dreams and the reality was she would never be mine. I felt an absolute fool. It's hard writing down in a book how I fell in love with a pop star, its something 13 year old girls do not a 25 year old bloke. Oh well I'm not afraid of making a fool out of myself that is for sure which is a good job I guess. I was firmly out of my fantasy land now but I was struggling. I was in close contact with my Psychiatric Nurse, Adrianne and I confided in her my true feelings. The calendar stall was fantastic at first and I enjoyed working with the public again plus they had a Rihanna calendar, it was ok for about 4 weeks then I started to be extremely over critical about myself. One problem I have is I go bright red when people try talking to me; it's a problem I have had from being young. It's such an annoying thing to happen, when the spotlight is on me I get really hot under the collar and then I start stuttering and go Red. When I was working on the calendar stall it reached a peak for me, someone would ask me the simplest of questions and then my whole face would turn Red. I still suffer with it now and it does cause me to shy away from certain social situations. I find I'm more confident in places that have lighting that isn't too bright. This way I can hide away and no one notices as much. Maybe a cave would be the best place for me to socialise. People often comment and say your going bright red? I think in my head *"yeah, don't you think I fucking know."*

So my outlook on life changed, I'd been high all summer then around September my mood levelled to a more normal level but now it was heading further down. I managed to keep going to work for the 3 days which I was supposed to work, even though I was struggling. I managed to hold out well and nobody really noticed that I was struggling as much as I was and hurting badly deep down.

My Dad's birthday was on the 29th November and he had arranged for a group of us to play golf at Lindrick Golf Club. I agreed to play but didn't really want to, I didn't want to be around people instead all I wanted to do was lock myself in my room and shut the world away, I just wanted to be in bed alone in the dark. But of course I didn't do this I just ploughed on and hoped that everything would be fine. We went back to the Yellow Lion after and had a family meal plus some of the golfing lads where there. I hated it and couldn't wait to get home, I remember thinking that everyone was having such fun and that I was the only one who wasn't. I don't think anybody really noticed apart from my parents. Other people may have just thought I was a little bit quiet. I don't think I realised myself how tough things were. Some of the feelings of dread and worthlessness represented themselves like they did in my first episode. That feeling came back in my stomach which is like butterflies but more intense and the fog descended upon me once again.

My Mum and Dad started to become concerned that I appeared depressed and my Mum emailed her concerns to Adrianne, so although I thought I was putting on a good front I couldn't have been hiding my true feelings very well. My mood fell lower and lower daily and I was starting to panic now, it was around the start of December. If my high in the summer was around 100 out of 100 then at this stage I was down to around 20. My whole life was just one big nightmare, I believed every aspect of my life was negative and I couldn't see any light at the end of the tunnel. I admitted my true feelings to my family and that I was struggling. I remember going round to see my Grandma and she rang my support workers, they were convinced it was all part of my recovery and it was all part and parcel of becoming well again, but my close family knew differently and realised how bad things actually were. I even asked Adrianne if I could have for some Citalopram (the anti-depressant I had taken before) as I knew myself that something wasn't right and that I was in fact depressed. The problem with mental illness is you can't see how poorly somebody is and sufferers don't always fit in with past models or have the standard symptoms. I believe I was one of those people. I had strong feelings of guilt from my rampage in the summer, I was struggling to come to terms with what I was thinking and saying and the extensiveness of my campaign was starting to dawn on me. The energy I put into my crusade in the summer had switched poles and now I would feel the fury in equal quantities. Guilt is a common symptom with depression but what was even worse was I did have things to feel guilty about.

My mood was falling all the time and by now it was about 15 out of 100, I was having disturbing intrusive thoughts and I couldn't shake them off and I was convinced that I was going to hurt somebody even though the truth was I wasn't but by this time I couldn't see the rational truth behind these awful thoughts. When I was poorly back in 2010 I had these awful thoughts and again when I was unwell now I couldn't see the truth. I believed that I was the person I was having in the thoughts. I remember seeing an old school friend when I was working on the stall and I got chatting to him, he was telling me how he had bought a house with his girlfriend and he was getting on well in his job. All of this became too much for me and I started having a panic attack, it started after he went. I think I just so badly wanted to do well in my life and it scared me hearing about everyone else's good news. I was always comparing myself to others and when you're nearly at rock bottom I always came off worse when making such comparisons. Comparisons are very dangerous. I often had panic attacks when I was working and my mood would be like the big dipper, one minute I would be ok the next I would swing wildly out of control in a downwards direction. This is known as rapid cycling in medical terminology (not peddling fast in a bike race) and when it was at it's worse it would happen many times in a day and I had no control over it.

My Grandma had seen an advert in the local paper advertising the Sheffield Bi-Polar UK group so she rang them up. It turned out that they had already had the December meeting and the next one wouldn't be until well into the New Year but they did inform her of another meeting which was the first Wednesday in the month in Chesterfield. I was in a right mess on the evening of the Bi-Polar meeting, my Mum and Dad had asked Adrianne to come round which she did and drew diagrams and gave me some breathing exercises to do to try and stop the feelings of panic that were coming over me in waves but all that was to no avail. Adrianne left some sleeping tablets for me to try and help me sleep as yet again I was not sleeping and hadn't done properly all summer.

I was at rock bottom and I was just totally distraught inside and I couldn't see any chance that this dark cloud would lift. I had aired my suicidal thoughts around this time. Mum, Dad, Grandma and I set off for the Bi-Polar meeting and I expected the meeting was going to be in a lecture hall type venue where there would be one speaker so I could just sit and listen and go home but it turned out to be in a smallish room with tables on one side full of crisps and snacks and biscuits as it was the last meeting before Christmas. There was a circle of around 20 chairs in the room and some people were already there when we arrived including Steve, who chaired the meeting. Steve has a great way about him and is fantastic at chairing meetings, he adds so much energy to a situation. On the night we attended we all went around in the circle and said a little bit about ourselves. Out of the four of us the circle got round to me first and I just explained how I was struggling with certain matters and was finding things difficult, if I had said exactly what was going on in my head they would have probably called an ambulance. My Grandma introduced herself and said she was my grandma and that we were here to try and understand and help. It was then my Dad's turn and he began saying we had all been through a terrible time and he let all his emotions out and was very upset, he just said he felt hopeless with it all and described everything that had happened before and just basically let go. This was good for my Dad as he isn't one for letting his emotions out. My Dad had an exceptionally tough time due to the total lack of support from his own family which must have added to his sadness. In fairness to my Nannan she was being told lies from Richard. Luckily my Mum's family and their friends supported him throughout the troubles and gave him the love he desperately needed to allow him to repair his broken pieces. No father should be the subject of what I did, I was told the torment behind closed doors was beyond belief. I guess the whole situation shows how strong my Mum and Dad are, if they can withstand the trauma of what I put them through then I'm sure they can survive anything. One of the members of the group came over and he gave my Dad a hug. I think the whole experience helped my Dad as later on he wasn't as upset and in fact he was very positive about my situation after speaking with other members of the group that night. My Mum was also upset and just introduced herself to the group as my Mum, she couldn't say anything else as she was very choked up. Afterwards they all went across the road to the pub and I got chatting to a few other members, I got chatting to a girl called Suzanne and she was very helpful and after speaking with her and a few other people I begun to feel up lifted like a massive weight had been taken from me. For the first time in months I felt like my old self. I thought I had cracked it, all I needed to do now was go home take my sleeping tablets and all would be well in the world. My Mum, Dad, Grandma and I got in the car to go home and we were all so pleased we had been to the meeting and felt that it had done me a power of good and there was just a general air of relief that I seemed to be feeling much better and I went home after the meeting feeling great. I remember thinking on the way home what had I been so worried about? What was I so frightened of as there really was nothing to fear. So I took the sleeping tablet and managed to get a little sleep but not a full night's sleep and before I knew it the thoughts were back and I was near rock bottom yet again. I remember getting up that morning and going to get a shower, my mood was very low and I had that feeling in my stomach. I got in the shower and for some reason when I got out I was feeling totally fine again, so much so I even rang Adrianne to tell her how much better I was and thanked her for all the help she had given me, my mood continued to stay high and I opened up the stall at the Calendar Club as normal but before I knew it the horrible feelings came back and I was feeling like shit again, the day on the stall was extremely turbulent and my emotions were all over the place. People from other stalls would come over to talk and I'd go bright red and not be able to talk back. Then all of a sudden I'd be totally fine again and I'd look back and think Christ what was I thinking. Then the whole cycle would repeat itself and I'd be back to square one. I managed to get through the day and went home with my Dad.

The next day I got up after another night of no sleep, I had already been downstairs at around 4am and had a cup of tea with my Ma. My Mum had come into my room and had tried to help me with my breathing exercises to relax me as I was breathless and was taking massive gasps of air but nothing was working. My whole body was trembling. The bad energy within me was so strong and I was so frightened but what of? All the bad thoughts were going through my head and I was having intrusive thoughts to hurt my Mum and at the time I, of course, believed that the thoughts I was having were actually true. Add in the fact that I hadn't slept for a week or so plus everything else that was going on inside my head including the fact that I felt I had no confidence in talking to people and that my whole life was going wrong. Then of course add in the guilt from the summer. The embarrassment from my wild fantasies and the fact that I had done everything so publically. I had no girlfriend, still lived at home plus had very little cash, no job and generally had an extremely low opinion of myself. All my close mates were the total opposite and I found that hard to take. I literally felt like I was a nobody. I just felt alone and that no one would understand what I was going through, the intrusive thoughts were the worst thing that I have ever experienced. They were worse than depression much worse and I was beginning to frighten myself. It's like there was a machine in my head playing out the same horrendous commands. Over and over again, they never left me.

Looking back now I can see that what was happening; I was still on my way down from the high I had in the previous summer. My chemicals were still adjusting and I was in the process of a balancing act. So here we are Friday morning with everything rushing through my head, I was very anxious, nervous and couldn't focus. All these horrendous thoughts were going through my head and I believed every one of them. It was awful to believe that I had the capacity to carry out these distressing thoughts. My Mum was off work as she was going on her Christmas day out with all her friends and she had said she would take me into work. She realised when we got up that I was in no state to go to work and said she would phone them up and explain and also she wouldn't be going out on her friends' day as she needed to get to the bottom of this. She made me a cup of tea and told me to go and sit down while she nipped out with our dog Billie for 5 minutes. The intense messages were playing out louder and louder in my brain, the thoughts were getting more intense and rapid. It felt like I was going to do something extremely bad to my Mum. It kept going, the thoughts just intensified. I knew I was going to do something, she would walk in any minute. What was I going to do? The messages kept being playing in my head. I was just pacing around. They were real, what was being said in my head was going to happen any minute. I was left alone in the kitchen and I went and got a kitchen knife from one of the drawers. I then went to cut my wrist but only slightly and it made a small cut, once I had made the first cut I then slashed my right arm 6 times, I knew nothing was happening so I put lots of pressure on my left wrist and made another 4 cuts. This time they were deep. As soon as I cut the left side my hand went numb.

I had to do something to stop the craziness inside my head, I just couldn't take it, it was the worst thing you could ever imagine. I just kept slashing my wrists, I needed it to go away, it didn't so I kept cutting until it did. Blood shot everywhere, it was just like somebody had shot holes in a high pressure boiler, it just went everywhere with great intensity and coverage. The feeling of slashing my wrists felt like I was scouring a piece of Pork. I realised I wasn't dying so I then got the knife and tried stabbing myself in the chest with the aim of going through my heart but it was too hard and I couldn't do it. Blood was pouring out everywhere, there wasn't a bit of our cream kitchen floor you could see as everywhere was covered in blood. My Mum was coming in the gate at the top of the garden and I just stood in the kitchen doorway and shouted

"Mum" ….. "I've cut myself look what I've done".

I think I was in shock and I just felt numb. It was like a scene out of a horror movie. Nothing mattered, I thought if I can't kill myself what can I do now? I so badly wanted to end my life that the pain of slashing my wrists was less than the pain of living. I attempted to end my own life as everything to me at the time was finished, my whole life seemed hopeless and the thing that tipped me over the edge and made me end my own life was the thought that I was going to kill my own Mother. I thought I had to kill myself in order to not kill her that's how real the thoughts were. How could I hurt the most precious person in the world to me?

I severed a tendon and a nerve on my left hand meaning my hand just curled up, my fingers on my left hand was, and still are, numb.

My mum ran up to me and grabbed my arms and put them above my head and told me to sit on the stool and not to move. She grabbed tea towels from the drawer and wrapped them tightly round my lower arms. She dialled 999 and was on the phone to the operator, keeping the phone under her ear with her shoulder she followed their instructions. They told her to unlock the front door and get towels and wrap them round the tea-towels on my arms and put tight pressure on them. She ran to the bottom of the stairs and shouted to my sister who was getting ready for work and told her to get towels quickly as I had hurt myself. My sister came down and obviously was in total shock and told me she loved me. There was blood everywhere and I mean everywhere. Both my Mum and Sister just kept a tight hold on one arm each and we must have been sat there a good 10 minutes before the ambulance turned up. I was just silent, I had nothing to say, nothing left in me, I was blank and empty, I was dead.

You may read this and think what a selfish person I am to do a thing like that knowing that my Mum and Sister would find me and in such an horrific state whether I be dead or alive. Some days I agree with that but as I look back and speaking to my family we all understand that I was very unwell. I just wanted everything to stop and the consequences didn't even feature in my head. I believed those intrusive thoughts and I thought I was capable of hurting my own Mother. That was like the worst thing I could think of doing, just like in the summer when I believed I was God, it was the complete opposite, my worst fear in the world, hurting my own Mum. That's what Bi-Polar is the two extremes of emotion, the high and the low. The ambulance turned up and they took off the towels my Mum had wrapped me up in and put on some temporary bandages. My Mum got me some more socks and put my shoes on and the ambulance women walked me to the ambulance. They then re-dressed my wrists and were concerned with the very deep cut on my left wrist. While this was all happening my Grandma arrived in her car, Christie had phoned her and asked her to come round. She arrived just before the ambulance left and came in the ambulance and gave me a kiss and told me she loved me then went into the house to see Christie. Can you imagine what it must have been like for them cleaning the kitchen, their brothers and grandsons blood everywhere? My Mum came and got into the ambulance and I was now in proper bandages and I don't think there was any concern for my life. They didn't put the lights on which of course I thought they would. The drive to the hospital seemed to last forever, we were bound for Rotherham Hospital which normally takes 10 minutes but on this day it seemed like half an hour. We arrived in A&E and I was put in a wheel chair at this point and they wheeled me into a room where they left just me and my Mum. We were there, again for what seemed like hours but in reality it was probably more like 40 minutes. I had nothing to say to my Mum, no sorry's, no tears, no nothing. I was still numb, not just my fingers but my feelings were numb. So we sat there, Mum trying to reassure me every so often, but basically in silence, I think I was still in shock with what I had tried to do and my Mum was too. I just did not know where to go from here, it was unimaginable. I was shaking and trembling and Mum just kept rubbing my back and saying everything would be all right.

We were called into a cubicle; the lady doctor was foreign and decided that my arms needed stitching. She stitched up my right arm totally but said she would have to leave my left arm as the cuts were too deep and I had severed a tendon and I would have to go to the Hand Clinic at the Northern General Hospital as it needed specialist treatment. So the stitches had been done on the right arm and my arms re-bandaged and I was then taken to CTR (Central Treatment Room) and told the staff what had happened and they arranged for the Crisis Team to come out to us in the Hospital. I was becoming increasingly paranoid, I thought they didn't mend my left hand as a kind of punishment for what I had done and that other staff were going to punish me.

So we waited in a tiny room for about an hour, by this time my Grandma had joined me and my Mum in this room just near A&E. After an hour or so two people turned up from the Crisis Team who are based at Swallownest Court, Rotherham. They interviewed me for about 30 minutes, I can't really remember what they were talking about but it was relation to my mental health and why I had done what I'd done. They said I would have to go back into hospital and asked if I would go voluntarily as opposed to being sectioned. I agreed and it was decided that I would go straight from the hospital in my Grandma's Mini with her and my Mum back once again to Swallownest Court Hospital.

I was checked in on the Osprey Ward at Swallownest Court, Rotherham on the afternoon of Friday 7th December 2012. I was taken with my Mum to a meeting room that was separate from the lounge and bedrooms. So here I was, arms bandaged up sat with my Mum and Grandma along with two young looking female doctors and a Nurse named Matt. We must have all been sat in this room for a good 40 minutes. I was interviewed about various aspects of my life including relationships, work, reasons for attempting suicide and if I had any plans to harm myself again. When they asked me why I done what I had done the only explanation was I believed I wanted to harm my Mum. My Mum stepped in at this point and explained that couldn't be true, but I was that adamant and no one could change my mind as I had heard these thoughts, they were real. So that's the explanation I came out with for my actions, I attempted suicide as I believed I would harm someone else. That's probably a fair description. The ferocity of what was going on within my head had frightened me beyond anything I knew was possible, what was going on in there was the definition of illness. Luckily for me the Consultant Psychiatrist Dr Cooper told me this was not real and they were just thoughts. The problem still was that I wasn't having any of it. The Doctors and Nurses were considering putting me in a close observation room on the Kingfisher Ward like I mentioned earlier, in the end they decided to leave me on Osprey. As I'd been there before I kind of knew what to expect from my stint in summer 2012 however things were very different this time. This time I was severely depressed and had just attempted suicide, whereas before in the summer I treated the place like a hotel and very few things phased me. After the interview with the two young doctors I was shown to my room. I took an instant liking to Matt, he was very calming and reassuring. In the interview the doctors asked about my driving and I explained that my licence had been taken off me and Matt told me that eventually I would get it back. I of course knew I would never get it back. That's just a small example of how he was always reassuring me, he told me that I would get better. At the time everything he or anyone else for that matter said meant nothing. Maybe somewhere deep down inside me their positivity actually sank in. Another special person from my stay in hospital in December 2012 was Shirley who was fantastic as I said previously when discussing my stay at Osprey in the summer. She took on the role of my mother while I was in hospital, I wasn't alone in receiving this comfort, all the other patients also did. However you didn't want to get on the wrong side of her as she would let you know just like she did on one occasion with me. When I used to talk to her I was always looking in my past and she said on numerous occasions *"Yesterday is history, tomorrow is a mystery and today is a gift and that is why we call it the present"*. So I was very lucky to have two very good contacts while I was in hospital. At the time though I couldn't see it, all I could see was one big mess, a black hole and darkness. I was just completely numb that's the only way I can describe it. So it was early evening when my Mum and Grandma finally left on that dreadful Friday. It was tea time soon after, but I wasn't allowed to have tea as I was supposed to be having an operation on the Saturday so no food was allowed. I was in a total dream world that night, twelve hours earlier I wanted to die and still did.

Now I was alive and in hospital. My room was right at the end of the corridor near the lounge so I was nearer the staff so they could monitor me more easily through the night. The checks at night are normally one per hour but on my first few nights they were more like every fifteen minutes. I spent that first evening in my room. I looked extremely sorry for myself, both my arms had thick bandaging on them and it was obvious to the world what I had done. I wasn't allowed to get them wet so I wasn't allowed to shower. My Mum and Grandma were back on the Saturday to pick me up to take me to the Northern General Hospital in Sheffield. I was very introverted and shaking badly all the time, my Grandma had put blankets in the car and I wrapped myself up in it but it didn't stop me shaking. We got to the specialist hand clinic at the hospital and it was packed out. I was sat there and I was convinced everyone was looking at me, in truth I don't think they were but given my state I wouldn't have blamed them. With it being my arms it was obvious what I had done and it wasn't very easy to cover them up. I remember thinking I wish I had taken an overdose as that way no one else can see. It's a horrible thought to have but I was in a bad place. I was sat in between my Mum and Grandma in the hand clinic for about three hours; it was then that my Mum found out it was too late to do operations by then. They called me in and my Mum followed, they told her that she couldn't come but she told them she needed to be there. They read my notes and it said what had happened and they allowed her to come in with me. A very nice nurse thoroughly cleaned my wounds and this involved a number of small injections around the wounds. They only looked at the left arm as my right one was stitched the day before at Rotherham Hospital on the day of my suicide attempt. I remember when the pain was bad thinking to myself; you're not a bad person. So maybe deep down I knew I was not a bad person? By now my paranoia had kicked in again as the nurse/doctors at Rotherham Hospital (where I first went on that Friday) had told us that you only get twenty four hours to mend the tendon and my twenty four hours were up, I believed that I was being punished for attempting to end my life for the impact it had on everyone around me. Anyway I was booked in for a few days later to have my surgery. By now I didn't believe I would ever get any movement back in my fingers.

Monday morning came and my Mum and Grandma came again to pick me up to go to the Northern General Hospital, I was still in a trance and shaking uncontrollably. Now time frames all merge in to one really. I recall seeing the doctor before hand and I was in a real bad way, my Mum had to tell them I wasn't well and suffering with Bi-Polar, I at the time thought she didn't really mean it and they were talking in code. What I thought she meant was he's putting it all on and there is nothing wrong with him. So the doctor asked whether I would like a local anaesthetic or a full anaesthetic, I wanted to go to sleep. I remember thinking maybe if I get put to sleep my body and life would reset itself and this whole living nightmare would go away, but guess what, it didn't! I woke up very fast from the surgery and I was panicking, I asked where I was and I seem to remember the nurse saying *"you're in hospital, you tried killing yourself"*, now I cannot be certain she said this as I wasn't all there but I do think she said that or possibly I was dreaming. I was very hot after the operation and they were concerned with how hot I had become. The good news from the operation was they mended the tendon and I was told I would get full movement back in good time but it would still remain numb. I went back to Swallownest Court, now with a pot on my left arm and the right in bandages. At first my hand was curled up and my fingers were in a ball like shape. I was given some finger stretches to try and increase the flexibility and over the next few weeks my fingers started to open up again.

I saw the doctor the next morning in hospital; it wasn't Dr Cooper but an alternative as he wasn't in. I was put on 20mg of Citalopram and he also increased my Olanzapine from 15mg to 20mg. I was back on the ward and I had my Mum and Dad coming every visiting time to see me. My Grandma would also come daily. Shortly after I had been given the 20mg of Citalopram, I suddenly became well, all my problems disappeared, my Mum came to see me when I was in this state of being "alright", I told her none of the bad things I was thinking were true and that I had no intention whatsoever in hurting her and that I loved her so much. It was funny, although I felt fine I knew deep down that I wasn't fit enough to leave hospital, even despite the fact that I was feeling perfectly ok. I said to myself at the time that I shall stay in hospital and I won't be leaving until the end of March. I don't have a clue where March came from.

This feeling of being well and not paranoid and not having intrusive thoughts soon disappeared, and I was back to where I was a few days before. As I was an informal patient (i.e.; not being held under a section of the Mental Health Act) I was able to leave the hospital when I wanted, however I never exercised that right. Maybe if I had tried to they would probably have sectioned me. I stayed on the ward for a week and on the Sunday my parents asked if I could come home for a bath, a friend of ours had given us some plastic covers for my arms so at last I was able to soak in a bath. My Mum and Dad picked me up and after speaking with the staff on the ward agreed I wouldn't be left on my own at all. They took me back to my Grandma's where I had a bath, got changed and sat and relaxed for a couple of hours and it felt great, my mood went from being really low and depressed like to a sense of relief that I wasn't poorly. However this didn't last long and my mood dropped again when it was time to go back to the hospital. I believed they had put something in my coffee so that I would feel good and then they would take it from me as some kind of torture. Again as I wasn't sectioned I was allowed to go home more frequently than other patients, at first I went home every other day for a couple of hours, then for tea but I wasn't coping very well and my head was all over the place. My two mates Richard and Tom came to see me I told them that I was going to hurt people and wanted to be sent to Rampton High Security Hospital, this was built on the fact that I was having so many disturbing thoughts. As time went on my intrusive thoughts got worse and worse and around this time I spoke with my Dad and told him that I wanted to go to Rampton. He told the staff and they stopped my leave. So here I was trying to convince people firstly that I wanted to hurt my Mum, then that I wanted to hurt other patients and then I wanted to end up in a high security hospital. They made me another appointment to see Dr Cooper and he agreed to increase my Citalopram to 30mg and the Olanzapine was left the same. Again after the increase my mood lifted and yet again I told everyone that the things I had been thinking weren't really what I thought and that the truth was I didn't want to hurt anyone. My leave was given back to me and I went home again for my tea, I stayed ok for about four days and the Doctor agreed to increase my leave to one overnight at home, so I thought this is great, I'm on the way out of here and I'm getting better. So I went home on the Friday and everything was great, I remember watching telly with my Mum and sister and we had loads of chocolates. Everything was going great, I went to bed and had a good nights sleep but woke up feeling worse than when I went to bed. I still wasn't too bad but my mood had dropped from the previous night. I went out with my friend Ben to B&Q and was managing to hold things together but I remember not having much conversation as my mind was elsewhere. But I got through the day; all I wanted to do was lie on my bed in the dark. So I went to bed the Saturday feeling not 100% and a little worried. I woke up the following morning panicking, I was having a panic attack, my breathing was really heavy and I couldn't focus. I don't have a clue why I woke up in this state; I remember picking my nose so hard I made it bleed, this was kind of a nerves thing. So I went to the bathroom and on the way saw my Dad, he asked what was the matter and I said I didn't know but I was having a bit of a panic attack. I calmed down a bit but I was feeling shocking again, my intrusive thoughts weren't back yet but I was getting very worried. I think I just didn't want the day light to come, I wanted the darkness to stay. I went that morning to watch Alex play football, all I kept doing was thinking how I wished I could be him, I would have been happy to be anybody else but me that's how rotten I felt. The thing that I was doing all the time was comparing myself to others. Given the fact I was in hospital and severely depressed meant I would never win. So I went back to hospital feeling very low and sat on my own in my room and stared into space. I didn't want to mix with the other patients, I didn't want to talk to anybody I just wanted to be left alone. It's really hard to describe how I felt. I felt empty, I was afraid, alone and desperately didn't want to be me anymore. One of the lads from the ward found out that I was informal and he used to ask me all the time to go to the shop, I of course didn't dare stand up to him and would always be having to go the shop. I thought this is a taster for what prison life will be like, I knew I'd get bullied horrifically as I didn't know how to stand up for myself.

It was Christmas week and all the staff were decorating the ward but I didn't feel like Christmas one bit. I was walking around like a zombie, I was given some Temazepam and diazepam to try and take the edge of things but it didn't really have a great deal of affect. I remember once just pacing around my room and there were a group of patients outside my window and one of them was a gentleman who was Indian. I was having really bad intrusive thoughts that were very racist and I was certain I was going to shout something to him as that's what my thoughts were about. Now the truth is I'm not racist one bit but I convinced myself that I was. It was then that I came out of my room as I was getting worried and saw Martin one of the nurses. I just started pacing around the living room like a man possessed and couldn't settle, it was then he prescribed the meds. Martin is another lovely nurse who is great at looking after people. All the staff at Swallownest Court were great. The ward manager Mark was also fantastic, I remembered him from the summer. In one of our long chats he said to me what do you want to do when you get out of here, I replied with I'm never going to get out. He then talked me into the idea that one day I would get out and eventually I told him that when I get out I want to go to this Turkish restaurant with all my friends. I often had chats with the nurses and nursing assistants, there were a few fitties too and I think bit by bit they made my life that little bit better but at the time it didn't feel like it.

Dad brought mince pies in for all the patients in the ward which they all loved, I too ate a lot of them as I was craving sweet stuff due to the Olanzapine.

The staff on the ward agreed that I could go home for my Christmas lunch so Mum picked me up around 12 noon and we went home. I stayed with my Grandma while they went for a quick drink at the local pub then we all had dinner together. The day was horrendous I'm afraid to say, I felt shocking and truth be told I had given up. My Mum and Dad had gone to so much trouble and to be honest I did feel a little guilty for not enjoying myself more. I tried my best though to not put a downer on the day but that only went so far and once again I had ruined things for my hardworking parents.

Christie took me back to the hospital around 8pm with Mum and I was very unwell. I just couldn't see any future or anyway out, I was extremely depressed and my mood was at rock bottom.

The next day was Boxing Day, originally I had been going to watch Rotherham United with my dad, brother and some friends, but I wasn't well enough so instead Mum picked me up with my Mums friend Rachel and we came home. In truth I just wanted to be kept alone and just left there but that was never going to happen. So I went back to my parents' house and we had tea but I just felt like a hindrance. It was hard to be around people who seemed to be having fun and enjoying themselves. That was just my perspective however they probably weren't due to me not being well. I just wanted to get out of the situation, when I was at home I wanted to be in hospital and when I was in hospital I wanted to be at home. Story of my life, I always want what I can't have. So all in all Christmas was a very tough time, not just for me but for everyone in the family. I'm not sure what my parents were thinking or how they saw an end to this. They had been assured by all the staff that I would get better but it wasn't happening and they were becoming ever increasingly concerned.

My Grandma would come down in the day to see me with a piece of chocolate flapjack from my favourite local bakers in Swallownest and a flask of coffee complete with milk (not for me) and sugar, she thought of everything and as always was well prepared for any occasion. My Mum and Dad would come in the evening to see me, they brought with them more goodies and always a bit of fruit. One time my Mum went to the effort to buy me some cakes and I told her I didn't want them. I thought they were trying to get me used to the sugar in my blood and once I was reliant upon it they would withdraw it to kind of punish me and make me suffer. My Mum was very upset when I told her not to bring me anything else, I felt very guilty but wanted to avoid the potential pain as much as possible. My Mum then went and changed her shift pattern so she could see me more. They wanted me to be alone in hospital for as little time as possible and that is something I look back on and am very grateful for. If I'm honest though I wanted to be left. My good friend Richard came frequently, I didn't like having many visitor's as I had nothing to say to them but I do appreciate the effort Richard put in and so do my parents. He'd just talk to me for a full hour and I would say nothing in return, when the time was up I'd hint that I wanted him to go. He and Tom arranged to go skiing and when he told me about it I just felt crippled, it felt like another body blow. Tom, Kidder and Matt also came sometimes. I was just ashamed of myself for a whole host of reasons and hated every fibre of my existence.

It was around this time that my family and more importantly my Dad had the sad news that our family dog Billie had lymphoma and there was nothing they could do to help him. I'm not a massive fan of dogs but I loved Billie to bits. He was the most beautiful looking Labrador I've ever seen. He had a thick Golden neck which made him look like a lion. He would walk with a slight swagger and had a Pink nose. On many occasions he would escape out of the garden and he would always head to the fields where he loved to play. No animal before or after has grabbed me like Billie. He had his very own personality and become my other Brother. In all fairness I didn't do a lot for Billie, Alex and Christie used to take it in turns taking him out and so would my Dad. But what I did do for Billie was love him and he knew that. I would take him out on occasions, more for my benefit than his. Before I became really unwell I used to take him into the fields, when I was down it used to temporarily perk me up been out with him. It gave me some purpose and reward. It was very therapeutic and he gave me something that no human could. Later on even when the carnage was going on in my head he would always come and lie next to my feet and if he could he would have put his arms around me to try and make everything better. He knew I was hurting. He will have found a big open field up there where he can wander all day without anybody wanting to bring him home. He will have found his home.

As it was Christmas a lot of the doctors were off on their holidays and it wasn't until the Monday after New Year that I saw the doctor again. I was very low and not getting any better and he increased my Citalopram to 40mg, this was the highest they would give me I was told. My mood lifted for a couple of days after Dr Cooper increased my Citalopram but this unfortunately was only temporary and I soon reverted back into my depressed state of mind. It was strange when my mood lifted because I remember thinking yes, this is it, I'm better, like I had done previously but unfortunately it wasn't to be. I just wasn't making any progress it was like one step forward three steps backwards. It was an awful time, words cannot describe how I felt, my world and life had been taken from me, I literally believed I was nothing and due to all these horrific thoughts I believed I was the worst of the worst. I met with the Hospital

Psychologist Ray and tried to say how I felt, the things I was saying were of an extreme bizarre nature. I told him I was more evil than anybody in history and nobody was beneath me. He tried to inform me that nobody is 100% evil. That's a debate for another time. But I insisted I was.

The lads in the hospital were all great including Tyron, Lee and Paddy. They were the people I used to speak on the ward but I kept myself to myself most of the time. Paddy was a great bloke and we often talked about land rovers and off roading and shared videos on YouTube. It's funny my mood always lifted at night time, I have my own theory as to why and that was I knew I was going to bed where it was dark and I was alone. I would always wake up and all my worries would rush back and the nightmare would start again for another day. On one of my up moments I downloaded Ben Howards Every Kingdom which was fantastic to listen too, most of the time I was too low to even listen to music I just wanted to stand and gaze into nowhere. When I listen to that album now it takes me right back to that observation room on Osprey where they had put me. I guess it's a stark reminder of how serious my condition is and how much I have to respect it. When I first saw Paddy he was in combats and looked like he had walked straight out of the marines. Put it this way you wouldn't want to mess with him. When he was first admitted I was very paranoid and unwell, so much so that I thought he was a prison officer from Rampton (the high security hospital I thought I was going to) he was put in the bedroom next to mine. He had a lot of charisma but had a lot of his own demons to deal with. I remember thinking why is a man like that in hospital and struggling when he has so much going for him and has such a way with people, he probably thought the same about me. I told him one night that I thought he was out to get me and he was totally shocked and couldn't believe what I had been thinking. Unfortunately Lee is no longer with us and it is a massive loss for everyone who knew him as he had a heart of gold but had major demons that he had been trying to fight for many years but the pain must have got too much for him. Another lovely gentleman was Nigel, he was a lot older than myself but acted as a fatherly figure to me during my stay and was very caring. I would spend a lot of time with Nigel and he has a lot to give to the world. I was on a bit of an up when Nigel was round so luckily he never really saw me at my worst.

Whilst I was on the Osprey ward something happened to me which made me question everything I knew and thought about life. A very poorly patient, who was an informal patient, came up to me and told me that he had been home and got a load of Benzo's. He told me he could no longer take the suffering and would take the pills that night. He made me make a promise not to tell a soul. I promised I wouldn't. Now my head was pretty messed up at this point anyway but this just took it to new extremes. I didn't know what the fuck to do. If I tell the nurses I break my promise, the patient kicks of at me and makes my life difficult on the ward and I deny him the right to end his suffering. But he does not die. Alternatively I do nothing, the patient takes the overdose and ends his life as he wishes, I receive no trouble on the ward, things remain simple and I stick to my word and keep my promise. However he then looses the opportunity to get well in the long run and his family suffer. I didn't know what on earth to do. How could I live with myself knowing that my actions or lack of actions would lead to somebody ending their own life. What would you have done? Rightly or wrongly I did nothing. I'll tell you why. I didn't have the balls to deal with the consequences from this man. He would have been extremely unhappy and given his frame of mind I wasn't sure what the consequences might have been. I thought about myself and myself alone. I came up with some bullshit moral reason for doing nothing but the truth was I didn't have it in me to cause friction. Given the same event occurring now I'm not sure what I would do. Your kind of playing god no matter what you do and I knew full well the consequences of doing that has. Life and death is in your hands. Luckily the patient didn't do anything which made my decision much more easy to live with. Things were starting to get pretty intense and things were happening that frightened me. People with mental health problems often have something deep within them which makes you question everything you believe and everything you stand for.

One of my up moments was around New Year 2012/13. Even though I was stuck in hospital and all my friends and family where on the outside I had one of the best New Year's I'd ever had. We all sat up and watched the fireworks on telly and we all had some Schloer which as you know is non-alcoholic. I was just pleased to be alive. It was great having these special people around who were genuinely concerned about my welfare, I could feel their warmth. It's good to know that there are good folks out there especially when you think of a stereotypical psychiatric patient. I was once told that it's usually the real good guys that suffer with mental health issues and given all the people that I met on my 3 admissions I can certainly agree with that statement. On a separate night we all sat up and watched One Flew Over The Cuckoo's Nest' which was a surreal experience to say the least. Unfortunately this good feeling didn't last and shortly after New Year I went down I kept going down and down until I couldn't get any further down and once I hit rock bottom I then had to work my way back up. The way my condition got worse was with the intrusive thoughts, once I thought I was murderer that wasn't bad enough, I'd then convince myself that I was a paedophile then from there the only place to go was upwards.

Dr Cooper introduced the idea of Lithium to me, he told me it can be a very toxic drug and explained that you have to go for blood tests every 3 months. At the time he initially told me I thought I don't want to go on Lithium as I don't want to have blood tests as I don't like injections, I failed to see the possible benefits. Given the possible benefits an injection 4 times a year is a small price to pay. When my mood was still artificially higher due to the recent increase in Citalopram I remember saying to everyone look at me now I don't need Lithium. This time when my mood went back down I went into an even worse state, the disturbing intrusive thoughts came back, but this time much, much stronger. I had other meetings with staff members and my parents and I decided that as nothing else seemed to be working I would give the lithium a try and so I had blood tests and began taking my new medication. I had blood tests everyday until my Lithium levels were at an optimum level.

Mick, one of the nurses, came into my room one day with a note pad and a pen, just before this I had been pacing about my room, my mind was all over, all these thoughts that I was having were true to me, I thought I was capable of really bad things. So Mick said what's on your mind Tom, I replied with *"Hell"*. I'd managed to convince myself that I was going to hell for all the bad things I had done and bad things I would possibly do in the future. I also told him that I was going to kill one of the patients and I told him I was a paedophile, given all this I thought I was going to Rampton. So to summarise I thought I was the worst person in the world, the total opposite from the summer when I was King. So Mick went away with his note pad probably a bit shocked at the things I was saying although in his job he was probably used to it. It was around this time I remember being on my knees in my room praying to someone for forgiveness. I'm not sure who I was praying too as who was out there that could help me? I spent every minute I could in my room, I wasn't talking to staff or patients I had just closed down. Following my meeting with Mick I had mentioned some of the things I was thinking to my Mum. She told me that I had to tell the staff everything I was thinking as this was the only way they could know how I was feeling and help me. Unbeknown to me my Mum and Dad were beside themselves and were despairing of the whole situation as they felt like my behaviour was similar to how I had been just before my suicide attempt back in December, even though I was taking all this medication. My Mum had phoned the hospital and spoken to the Head of the Mental Health Department and told him her fears and worries that I was not improving at all. At the same time I decided to come clean with the doctor about my thoughts, there is a database system where staff put notes on and they update it daily so that when you are due to see the Doctor he is able to be brought up to date before the meeting. The upshot of the meeting with the doctor was that I was to lose all my leave and he put me on Level 2 observations. This was because once again I had become a risk to myself. I think it was a wise move because at one point I had my belt strapped around my neck and wanted to pull it tight but couldn't physically do it. Yet again I needed out and that was the only way. I think I was just so desperate that I would have tried to do whatever to get out of this mess and now there was no hiding the doctors knew what I was thinking and they thought I was a risk to myself. At this point I had probably been taking Lithium for roughly 4 weeks. On Level 2 Obs (highest level) you have a member of staff within an arm's length of you at all times. I had been put on level 1 observations previously but improved and got taken of it when my mood temporarily lifted with the medication increases. With Level 2 Obs somebody even has to stand next to the toilet whilst you went in and the same for showering. They took my belt, shoe laces, phone charger and anything with a cable off me and I was put back in the observation bedroom where I had been a few weeks previously when I was on level 1 observations. At night I had to have my door wide open and the staff had to sit outside, it was a very bright corridor plus the room was next to the lounge so sleeping was very difficult. So I was with a member of staff twenty four hours a day. Given the fact I was on a one to one I had to talk to the staff. This made me release things from within my mind and get things of my chest, at first I was still extremely poorly. I told all the staff about my thoughts including the desire to go to prison and the fact I was a paedophile. One of the nursing assistants looked me dead in the eye and said *"are we safe Tom?"* I didn't know the answer but once I thought I'd convinced the staff that what I was telling them was true I started to panic a little. I then realised that maybe it wasn't me.

I asked for a one to one meeting which I had with Andy on the 13th February. He told me very bluntly that he didn't believe any of the things that I was saying and that none of it was true. For some reason this registered with me and suddenly this house of cards I had built with all the intrusive thoughts and belief systems collapsed slowly one by one and I then realised I wasn't this bad person that I was making out to everyone I was. Just like in the summer when I got the feeling of love back for my family and the sense of reality back. Some staff put my sudden jolt back into reality down to the fact that the Lithium had reached its optimum level. I do agree with that but it's also down to the fact that I put all my problems out there in the open and got everything of my chest, then once it was out there something changed which meant I no longer believed the horrible thoughts I was having before. I had released them from the vault and was the able to view them for what they were – thoughts. This process was only made viable due to the introduction of Lithium I believe.

When I commenced the Lithium programme, it meant starting on a very low dosage. I started on 200 mg then had blood tests and a week later my dosage was increased. My optimum level was 1000 mg and it took me 5 weeks to get to this point. I still have to go and have a blood test and attend the Lithium clinic once every three months.

So here I was feeling my normal self totally, all the intrusive thoughts had disappeared, well they never disappear but I could rationalise them rather than catastrophizing them and I felt the most normal I had felt in a year but I was still on the Level 2 Obs which meant staff still had to be with me at all times until a doctor had seen me which wouldn't be until the following week. I was an informal patient who was under close observations. This was something the ward hadn't come across before as normally anyone under close observations was under a section. I remember staff asking me on a number of occasions if I would leave the hospital if the door was opened and I replied *"no because I need to be in hospital"*. This was the right answer; if I'd have answered differently they would have had to section me for my own safety. In practice it wouldn't make any difference if I was sectioned or not but it just kept things simpler if I wasn't. Before I became better I was haunted by some of the people I had abused in the summer. For example I would sometimes see my hostages floating around plus the women I wasn't very nice too on the day of my tribunal. I apologised to her, I guess like in life I was paying the price for my actions in the summer. What goes around comes back around.

While I was in hospital I had a few people from the bi-polar UK group come and see me, namely Steve and Andy. Both didn't drive so they had to get buses and trains over from Chesterfield. They were a great support and Andy even brought me loads of chocolates. Their visits were fantastic and I still keep in touch with them. It was nice to be around people who had suffered and understood. Both Steve and Andy had been hospitalised previously and knew what I was going through although nobody unfortunately knew how bad the intrusive thoughts were. Nobody I spoke too had had such thoughts to harm others. I see Andy regularly and he is a great support and offers fantastic advice.

Gradually overnight visits were recommenced and by Monday 11th March, just over 3 months after my suicide attempt and admission into hospital I was discharged from the Osprey Ward.

33. BACK INTO SOCIETY

I felt like I had swam the channel, my mood when I left was right in the middle not too high and not too low, as fellow bi-polar sufferer and support worker Jason says, *"keep your legs above the shit and your head below the bullets"* meaning just stay in the middle. I just couldn't believe the journey I had been on since the summer of 2012 right through to the events of the winter. I felt like I had gone full circle and maybe I was off the merry go round. Who knows the answer to that? Nobody I'm afraid. It's a fear that hangs around your neck, some days I feel as free as a bird and nothing worries me, other days I sometimes feel a bit off and believe that maybe the illness is creeping its way back into my life. But like I said at the beginning, the illness is with you for life, there is no operation to rid you of this disease. On the whole I have been on a very even keel since the end of February 2013 but I've had a few wobbles along the way.

In addition to my release, my nephew Theo James was born on 13th March 2013. It was very timely and coincided nicely for everyone as the family was in a position to divert some much needed love and attention to my brother and his new family. Nicole is a fantastic mother to Theo, she is a natural and has a great connection with him. Working with children is definitely her vocation.

Over the last few years I had soaked up my families love and time and it was time to reduce my requirements and redistribute it. Theo is an absolute treasure and gives us all so much joy, I guess he takes after his uncle in this department.

Once I was discharged from the hospital my care was transferred to the Home Treatment Team who called regularly the first week whilst I was home. I had weekly meetings with Adrianne and completed an Advance Statement. This is a document that I have signed while of sound mind which assists in my ongoing care and treatment in case I become ill again and of unsound mind. It includes signatures of my care co-ordinator and my consultant and the signs and symptoms that show if I am becoming unwell. It sets out what I would like happen to me and what medication I need to take and that all my other wishes about my home, children (if I have any) and my finances are to be dealt with by my parents and if for any reason I have to have a tribunal that my parents are to be present. It can be updated at any time I wish if my circumstances change. It felt strange writing out this document because you are pre-empting becoming unwell and the distress that brings with it. It was like signing your life away, because if it is ever used it means I have lost my mind again. Like everyone I just want to stay well and the content of the document was quite scary however it was something I had to do not just for myself but also the loving people around me. Similarly this book will also assist in helping me, if I do loose it again then in theory I can read this and realise that what I am thinking isn't real whether it be taking over the world or convincing myself I'm some horrific evil person.

Some of the things I believed perhaps mean, in some people's opinion, I should be incarcerated and fed medication to change what my mind is thinking. The truth is I am already caged in so have little to loose.

When I was out of hospital I returned to the monthly Bi-Polar UK meetings that happen on the first Wednesday of every month. It was good to be amongst people who were suffering with the same illness, there were usually about 20 or so people at the meetings and all had very different forms of Bi-Polar. Some people would become ill much more frequently than myself and really were quite poorly but not poorly enough to be in hospital. My type of Bi-Polar is one where I'm either ok or very poorly, I've had 3 episodes as you know and these have been very severe episodes where I totally lost track of reality on all 3 occasions. I often come away from the meetings feeling very fortunate as my illness is under control and is not controlling my life like it is for some other people. Maybe other Bi-Polar sufferers don't have the same support at home, maybe they didn't get the right treatment, maybe they are on the wrong medication or maybe they have a different type of illness. There are so many variables that contribute to the end result which in this case is how you feel. Some people maybe just give in and let the illness defeat them and become a victim. On the Stephen Fry documentary I watched on TV it said something like 20% of Bi-Polar sufferers go on to lead extremely good lives. I'm not sure what constitutes a good life but some people end up using the mental health services as a revolving door and never get out and I find that very sad and damaging. One thing I would like to get out of this book is reducing stigma. Before I became unwell I used to think that people with depression should just pull themselves together and get a grip, but when I was at my darkest moments there was no chance that I could sort myself out and shake it off and I am one of the most determined people I know. I was like many other people and didn't believe in depression before I was knocked down by it. I hope that people get help quicker and diagnoses are made sooner. Being diagnosed Bi-Polar has given me a sense of purpose and I'm no longer ashamed to tell people that I have it, however I think Manic Depression sounds better, it's less commercial. When I tell people they often don't believe me or comment that they would never have guessed. I guess it's because people think that people with Bi-Polar are either sky high or at rock bottom. Often people with no diagnosis have more symptoms of suffering from the illness, we all know someone who is either very happy or very sad. In my case I'm not like that and now I have a diagnosis and have found some medication that works for me I'm a very boring sufferer of Bi-Polar which for me and everyone around me is great but it's not good for any future writing material.

I've done a lot of work with my Psychiatric Nurse, Adrianne, we often talk about putting too much pressure on myself to fit in, this was a common theme running through my Cognitive Behavioural Therapy that I did with Claire. I so badly wanted to be this person and become this hypothetical individual that the more I tried the further I drove myself away from my goals. I read another good book called the Happiness Trap and this basically talks about allowing room for the problems in your life rather than trying to fight them. It says it you find space within yourself for the negative feelings then you are not fighting them and by doing so you, in theory, reduce the feelings of discomfort. It's very hard though, I always wanted to live a life that was absolutely free of negativity, so I was always fighting those feelings. I believed to be happy you were 100% positive with no bad feelings. Once I kind of accepted that things aren't always great then I became more at peace with myself. It's a very hard theory to put into practice and like most things worth doing requires practice. For instance I had some bad news about a job I had recently and before I would get all negative and create this massive friction between the bad feelings and myself and try to fight them away. What I did instead was say 'look this is a pretty shitty situation but I've just got to accept things for how they are'. This is apposed to taking on the attitude of 'why me?' The bad feelings don't go away they just become less noisy.

I didn't do anything exciting after leaving hospital, I just took things very steady. I still haven't had a drink since that awful night back in February 2012. It's not advised to drink a lot of alcohol whilst on Lithium as it dehydrates you which can lead to toxication. This suits me as I have learnt to live a good life without my old friend. I believe even without the Lithium I would still not be having a drink, I feel it keeps me much more in the middle and at peace with the world. It used to kill me though seeing all my mates going out drinking and going on all day benders but I'm way above all that now, I have as much fun now than I ever did, plus its real. Although I don't have that release from the daily grind and the feeling of freedom that a drinking session gives you, I have my health which is the main thing and more importantly, for the time being, my happiness. Who knows what my views will be in years down the line as I'm not sure what my attitudes will be then as we don't know what life is going to chuck at us. Truth be told I don't think I could deal with the hangovers plus everyone around me wouldn't be happy if I was to start drinking again.

I did a few odd gardening jobs over the summer of 2013 but nothing too stressful, I wasn't really too interested anymore in gardening and I still felt rather worn out, I enjoyed cutting grass but found other jobs like too much like hard work. I wanted to keep in my safety zone and turned a good bit of work down if it was too difficult and a bit of a challenge. I did however bite off a bit more than I could chew on the odd occasion and I had to get my old mate Richard to come to the rescue. If it would have been in the summer of 2012 then I would have been raring to go and wanted all the work possible but nowadays I'm a lot less driven and prefer to just chill out and listen to the radio, after all I did tell Mike I was retiring back in 2012. I am hoping to see my Physiatrist in the not too distant future where I'm hoping he will reduce my Olanzapine. Hopefully that will increase my energy levels but I have to be realistic. They gradually took me of the Citalopram when I came out of hospital and I still take 1000mg of Lithium. I am to stay on the Lithium for anything between 3 and 5 years and I've heard that when you come of the Lithium there is a strong chance you will relapse. One negative side effect of Lithium is that it makes you numb and you don't have as many feelings for things. Fortunately I'm not affected in this way. I have however put a great deal of effort into my book over the summer and also in maintaining my good health which takes up a lot of my resources at the moment. I think in time my drive and determination to succeed will return but at the moment I am just enjoying 'being'.

At the moment I don't have a great deal of energy to do anything other than work, the doc seemed to think that by maybe slowly reducing the meds this will help me however I cannot adjust the Lithium for some time. I was fortunate that the sun was shining for most of the 2013 summer time which allowed me to not only do a few jobs but also get out and about with my Grandma. We went to some lovely places and had some nice lunches out in various villages in Sheffield and the Peak District and also visited a few National Trust sites such as Haddon Hall. I really enjoy visiting the

Peak District especially on a nice summer's afternoon, even if it's just for a drive I still love it. I've been to some lovely places all over the world but nothing really feels as special as the peaks. I got my licence back on Saturday the 14th July which helped me with my ongoing recovery as it allowed me to get back into work and allow me to spread my wings and get away from the house. The good weather continued all summer and I continued to build on my recovery, there were a few ups and down but nothing like it had been. I even managed to go on a mission to Ibiza with my good friend Kidder. He was a great support throughout my problems, we had a fantastic time, saw some great DJs but we were disappointed as our friend Armin wasn't playing due to the arrival of his child. We watched a lot of beautiful sunsets in some secret hideaways away from the crowds. He's a right character is Kidder and has recently set up an electrical engineering company and I'm sure knowing him he will be very successful. He hopes to one day get a racing snail which if it's fast enough, he says, he will enter it into competitions. He's in my inner circle of friends. It was hard going away and staying sober however I knew I couldn't get back on the drink as it would have continued when I got home. I struggled with parts of the holiday as I wasn't used to mixing with strangers as I had just been in my safety zone for such a long time and still had major issues in mixing and talking to people plus I was still recovering. Kidder on the other hand was getting stuck in and certainly made up for me. I just didn't have any confidence in talking, I really wanted to be left alone. I think deep down I would have loved to have been going up to everyone and chatting but it wasn't the right time plus I felt very drained, possibly due to the meds or maybe just what my brain had gone through. I'd just been through some major life changes and was still trying to discover who I was. It was like I was starting over.

Shortly after arriving back from Ibiza I applied for a full time job at a company called Capita which is based in Wath, Rotherham. Capita is a customer services outsourcing company and many big firms use them. I went along for an interview as one of my friends has worked there for some time. I got all suited and booted and went along for the interview and they offered me a job there and then working for British Gas. I worked there until very recently. The training was very difficult and I struggled with it, this was mainly down to the fact that my brain wasn't used to absorbing information. Plus I had given it so much hammer over the last few years that it just wasn't working as well as it once did. We had 2 weeks training and then we started on the unit (where the phones are). It truth be told I wanted to pack in just a few days into the training, but I didn't. It's not a difficult job really however I found it tough, there is a lot of stuff to take in and the systems take some getting used too. I was hoping it was just a stepping stone into something else more in line with what I want to do however I don't really know what I want to do. I did want to work with young people who are going through mental health problems like I had or arguably still have but I found it very difficult to get any work. I considered applying to do Mental Health Nursing at University but later decided against it.

I decided to leave British Gas as I hated it and it was getting to me. The last thing I needed was sending backwards. I made some fantastic friends while I was there and they were the only thing keeping me going. However I thought that maybe my well-being was starting to become threatened and I decided to call it a day. I managed to squeeze in a trip to Cancun for Spring Break which was a fantastic week and my first American venture, me and Tom went with a few friends and Anthony who is not only a good friend but also the biggest boozer in Sheffield. Sometimes when he's on a big session he goes out and has 5 pints. He's also a bit of a ladies man.

Upon my return to Blighty I only had another week off and then I saw an advert for drivers at a firm locally, I had previously wanted a driving job however once I had an informal chat the owner, who was called Sam and was a lovely gentleman, he told me it was a sales role and it was all commission and no basic plus you had to pay for your van and ice. I would be selling frozen meat and fish door to door. All my mates and family told me it would never work but that gave me the drive to succeed. However after 2 weeks I decided it wasn't for me and I gave the van back. Sam was very supportive and kind towards me but I just didn't want to be selling door to door long term, the lads down there earn a great living from it but there different to me. At least I will never look back and think I wonder if I could have made it as a door to door sales man. Its very sole destroying when you knock on hundreds of doors and get no sales. One story I do have from the job was I accidently went to Van Persie's house in Alderley Edge. The big gates onto his housing estate opened as I approached them and I thought this is great they're letting me in. So I drove up the main drive then took a slight left turn onto one of the houses drives. I started to drive down the drive and a Range Rover was reversing so I reversed my Fiat Doblo off the drive and waited. I wound my window down and asked this man who I didn't have a clue who he was if he would be interested in any fish or meat, he was rather shocked and said bluntly that he didn't. His girlfriend started to have a go at me and said that I have to leave immediately and that I shouldn't be there, she said if I didn't leave the gates would close and I would be stuck there forever. As I said I didn't know the guy from Adam but he looked pretty cool and he had a Manchester United training top on so I googled Man U players and there was the man from the house on my phone!! So there we have it I tried selling meat to Van Persie! I also accidently stumbled upon Sir Chris Hoy - I think he accidently opened his gates after I rang the bell so I drove in again thinking great hopefully I'll get a sale as usually when people let you in their gates you tend to make a sale. However not Sir Chris, he certainly wasn't happy to see me. I didn't know him either but I knew I recognised him from somewhere and actually believed he was a chef, after searching on Google for a bit in my van I found him too! If I knew it was him I would have told him all about my spinning classes.

After leaving the sales role I started a temporary position in a pallet trading company based in Rotherham, here I worked in the transport office and dealt with their admin. The job was fantastic and I really enjoyed it and was pleased to have found something that I actually enjoyed. I was working hard and seemed to be getting to grips with it. I thought they would offer me a full time contract at anytime. My manager called me into the kitchen and I thought they must want to give me a permanent position. It wasn't to be, it turned out they wanted to terminate my contract and they gave me a weeks notice. I was gutted to be honest, I'd finally got to a settled point in my life and yet again something else was put in my stride. The company was going through a strange time and it was trying to double its share of the market in 5 years. This had created a lot of friction within the company and a lot of people weren't happy there. I don't think there really was a position for me, I believe I was just drafted it due to politics. I worked there for 3 months.

So here we are, the present and right now I'm just treading water, I can't seem to find a job that I can stick too and I so badly just want to find an occupation where I can flourish and progress. I wish the story had a fantastic ending where I had gone onto great things however as Baz Luhrmann says *"sometimes your ahead sometimes your behind, the race is long"*. So I guess something will come along at the right time and find me, but try telling me that. Part of me would love to go back to University and study Economics but what would I do with an Economics degree? Maybe I wouldn't even be able to complete the course again.

My friends often comment that I'm in a dream world and that I never remember things. The truth is I am, I have that much floating around in my brain that I surprise myself sometimes that I manage to function relatively 'normally'. Often my world is much greater than this world and I try my best to go there as much as possible. Likewise I often am sent to the darker side where its not so nice. I bite my nails too sometimes and people comment on this and say why do you look so nervous? Well I guess there's no real answer to that, I guess the future provides me with the greatest unrest. I've made peace with my past and kind of just get on with the present. If people knew what went on in my head they would be much more understanding and maybe forgive me for my distance with the real world. Sometimes people catch me talking to myself and find this rather strange or amusing, often I feel I am the only man in the world who can understand me or can explain the things that go of in my head. Sleep is my biggest worry as I often have a lot going on in my head and its difficult to switch it off. Lack of sleep in the past has been a major contributing factor to me becoming unwell and is the main signature of my relapse.

My wing man, Tom, has temporarily returned from the shadows after his relationship sadly came to an end. This is of course was great news for me but we both fully agree that we need to grow up and find some nice decent wife material. We have tried this but so far the results are not great. Of course the clock is ticking and if I don't find something soon I will be walking down the aisle with some random object. Both myself and Tom along with Sam, Ben and Anthony have re lighted the OTWC flame and get out on our bikes most weekends and a week day if we can. We've been on a great trip recently and we get a lot of fun out of those machines. I decided to loyal to Honda.

34. UNTIL NEXT TIME

If you open your eyes wide enough you too will see things that you didn't know where there and the answers to all your questions will become clear, things will happen and you will start to piece together your own little jigsaw unique to you, you will then be able to witness first hand your very own Masterplan. You just have to ask yourself, are you prepared for what you might see?

There is no truth in the world only your own, you only believe what you want to believe. This means anything is possible, there are no boundaries or limits. The answers are all out there, whether it is in films, songs, books, poetry, adverts, cloud formations, street names the list goes on. Everything that happens to you is not by fait, there is a underlying motive to every action within the universe. Once you put this book down you will start to see for yourself. Just remember to respect the system for you shall never beat it. Be careful, remember what happened to me.

My life could have been a lot different, I could have simply just accepted the conflict that was going on in my head and not question the world. That way I probably would have settled down with a girlfriend who maybe wasn't totally right for me, we'd probably be married now, I'd have an average job earning £22,000 which I wouldn't enjoy but it would help pay for my car that I'll never own and pay my mortgage which I really can't afford, I'd contribute to a pension and most likely have life insurance. I'd go to the pub on a Friday night with my friends around 7pm and arrive home at 10pm after consuming 5 pints and if I was feeling a little adventurous I'd have a packet of salt and vinegar crisps. I'd get up early on a Saturday and wash both our cars inside and out then I'd go and play football with my pals where I'd play midfield, I wouldn't be the best player but I'd be a valuable member of the team and I'd feel wanted. I then may call in the pub for 1 pint then go home to see the Mrs. We'd probably chat some bollocks about some bollocks then we'd cook a meal, no red meat and plenty of root vegetables. Sundays we'd get up really late, like 8.30am. We'd then go for a walk in our park, maybe wave to somebody we don't really know. Then I'd go round to the in laws who if truth be told I hate but she cooks a nice Sunday roast so it doesn't really matter. I would then proceed to drink 2 bottles of wine to try and make myself feel better and numb the pain. Plus hide the feeling that I would be going to work tomorrow for another 5 days of grind. O and the fact that I will repeat this process for approximately the rest of my life.

I on the other hand chose, well what did I choose? It arguably isn't life. But I've made my bed and I'm most certainly going to lie in it. I'm playing the long game however I never anticipated it to be this long. Sometimes in life you have to sacrifice being something to become someone. I might be remembered for a lot of things but I know one thing for sure, I dared to dream and big I dreamt. But dreaming doesn't get you very far unfortunately as I've learnt. I don't have a lot of the things you are deemed to need i.e. partner, money, house, flash car, career but I have something deep within my heart and soul that cannot be quantified and if for the rest of my days I only have that then I will die a happy man.

The fear never goes away, the fear that the good feeling inside disappears and possibly never returns. Like I say, this is chronic and for now there is no known cure. I just hope and pray that I can stay to live and fight another day. For when I'm gone what shall remain, a man who had a disease of the brain? I maybe insane but I no longer carry any shame. I hope more much more will live on, a legacy not a travesty.

I have latterly tried to treat life as a journey, for the destination is death. Once upon a time I used to try and make everyone happy and put their happiness before my own. Now I just focus on one person.

I guess it might be time to try and blend into the 9-5 life and get married to a girl who isn't totally right for me and possibly get a dog. Then again maybe I'll just stick to my guns. I know one thing though I don't want to be defined by mental illness. I most probably would have had a similar life without having a diagnosis of manic depression. It is no excuse for my past nor a prediction of my future.

One thing I would like to achieve from this book is helping one person who is going through a tough time. I would then like that person to help another person and so on. This is known in Economics as the multiplier effect and has the potential to create the most amazing results. Just like in the pyramid schemes, eventually your little initial investment can send ripples of strength to the people who need it the most, eventually these ripples get much bigger and stronger until one day they become great waves.

I wish I had more confidence in public speaking as I'd love to go into schools and other organisations and help promote mental health issues and raise the awareness as I feel if people weren't so frightened about the subject then people would be more open with their problems. This way issues could get nipped in the bud before they develop into a full blown psychotic episode which can lead onto other problems. Let's face it I should have died on the bridge in October of 2010 or if I planned my attempt in December 2012 I may have been more successful in slitting my wrists, luckily for me I'm not a great planner and my lack of preparation most probably saved me. It's just by luck rather than judgement that I've managed to stay alive. Maybe I wouldn't be sat here telling you my story instead I would just be another suicide statistic, not everybody gets a second chance and even fewer a third, I have been blessed by something throughout my journey and I am eternally grateful. I should have been treated correctly in the summer of 2012 then the low wouldn't have been so damaging, it's all about damage limitation. If I would have known the symptoms of my illness earlier then maybe I would have just kept myself well and avoided all the pain and torment not only for myself but also my close family and friends and most of all my parents.

I still of course have my scars and every day I see them and every day I'm taken back to that awful day. I can't escape it, I've got them for life and everyone who sees them knows what I've done, but hopefully one day people will understand more about why I did what I did. I always wanted tattoos but I guess I've got my own unique set of sleeves.

If you only get one thing from this book I would like it to be this;

No matter how hard life is, how dark things are, how lonely you feel or how much of a failure you perceive yourself to be. You will get through it, not only will it pass but by going through such pain you will not only be a better person but a tougher one too. So the next time that storm comes you know how to navigate your ship through it. As each storm comes and goes so does your ability to handle the rough seas. Just like in the real world, storms never go away for good. But the more you learn about yourself the easier it is to predict whatever adversity may be coming your way and the faster you will be able to take action. Never ever forget, you will get through it.

I owe a lot to the NHS and the British Government for funding my treatment, I thank science for the development of medication that has helped put my life back into some kind of order as without it I dread to think what existence I would have – if any. The hard work from the doctors for learning their trade also means not only I but many other people get the help needed. As well as doctors I owe a lot for the troops on the ground, the nurses, the support staff and all the people behind the scenes. After all no plane flies without good engineers, that is unless my friend Ben has anything to do with it.

I also thank the system for providing me with the financial aid throughout my difficulties in the way of Hospital Treatment, Ongoing support, Disability Living Allowance, Employment and Support Allowance, Housing Benefit, Job Seekers Allowance, Council Tax contribution, Working Tax Credits and other benefits I have received. I owe the system greatly not only for the financial assistance I have received but everything else. I intend to repay every penny I have taken out and restore the balance like all my previous debts. The system has worked for me but I learned very quickly how to play it and how to act to get the most out of it. A lot of people do not have the knowledge and insight when it comes to the system. People get let down by the system daily and although my story may give hope to some there are a 1000 bad stories to every story like mine. There were times when I was let down and there were failings I don't deny that but I'm a lucky kid. So many aren't. Sometimes people's faces just don't fit.

I am so fortunate to have such an amazing family and that has been commented by everyone who knows me from the hospital, my psychiatric nurse and my friends at Bi Polar UK.
I wear my Bi-Polar badge with pride and I feel we are the special ones. I went from believing I was King of the World to then believing I was the most evil person in the world, capable of murder. It's unbelievable how powerful the mind can be and how I could believe these two extremes of mood. I continue to take the meds every night without fail and I owe so much to the chemicals that are now in my brain. I'm not sure what might happen if I stopped taking them, maybe the King would return. Maybe I stopped taking them to write my book. That you will never know, I've told you most of my secrets but not them all. I have a long way to go before I can relax and take stock, I'm in an amazing place but there are still goals I need to achieve. Although I have very little interest in football I would love to see Sheffield Wednesday win the Premiership, yeah I guess I am still a little bit deluded in many ways. I'm a very ambitious person and I hope one day I can channel that ambition and create something amazing.

So that's my story so far - I only have one thing left to ask you:

"Do you think I'm crazy?"

Tom Gray

TOO FUCKING RIGHT I AM

Tom Gray

Lightning Source UK Ltd.
Milton Keynes UK
UKOW04f2353190615

253798UK00001B/4/P